LIVE OR DIE

A STROKE OF GOOD LUCK

by Richard L. Burns

Copyright @ 2008 by Richard L. Burns

Published by d&n Books, Carmel, CA 93923
www.liveordieburns.com

Distributed by Atlas Books, Ashland, OH 44805
www.AtlasBooks.com

First (Test Market) Edition co-published by Redwood Writers (California Writer's Club) and U.P. LLC, February, 2008

International Edition published March, 2010
Third Edition published February, 2012

Cover photography by Mike Sugrue, Sausalito, CA 93965 and Cover Art designed by BookMasters, Inc. Ashland, OH 44805 Subtitle phrase, "New and Improved" was originated by Procter & Gamble in 1946, changed numerous times and used by various products and many business and consumer publications.

ISBN: 978-0-615-52036-0

Library of Congress Control Number: 2012932347

LIVE OR DIE
A STROKE OF GOOD LUCK

by Richard L. Burns

To Nancy, wife, partner and friend who so patiently supported and guided; to Cy, selfless and wise physician who administered and counseled and to Gil who helped me put it all together.

TABLE OF CONTENTS

PART ONE

PART TWO

Live or Die
A Stroke of Good Luck

Foreword

Numerous books have been written about stroke, from both the stroke survivor and caregiver points of view, and I have read many of them. I have found that like snow flakes, each story is truly unique. I have also found that many of these stories have one common and powerful message—the message of hope.

In many ways, stroke is in its infancy. The verticals of stroke prevention, treatment and recovery are yet to develop in a way that allows significant progress to be made in the areas of public awareness or reducing incidence rates. Yet, stroke has been around for a very long time. Hippocrates is credited as the first to describe the sudden paralysis often associated with stroke, as being "struck down with violence". That was in 400-something B.C.

Fast forward to 1996, when the first-ever treatment for stroke received FDA approval. Imaging and diagnostic tools for stroke have advanced greatly in recent years and hospitals across the country are developing stroke centers, thereby incorporating stroke systems of care. Rehabilitation and recovery methods are improving. Hence, for the first time in the history of stroke, we have accomplished more in the past decade than ever before. Yet, we have much more to do. The Baby Boomer generation is now in the prime of their golden years and some say a tsunami of stroke could hit as this generation continues to age. Perhaps even more alarming is that stroke has become more prevalent among our younger population. All of this history is why it is more important than ever that we continue to spread the word about stroke. Everyone in the U.S. deserves to know how to recognize and respond to warning signs, to understand what stroke really is and how it affects survivors and their families. There is much to be learned from the more than seven million survivors in this country. What better way to carry these messages than through the real-life stories of those that have lived it?

This is a story of one man's journey down the lifelong road to recovery. It provides yet another inspiring example of the will to reset the clock to a life before stroke.

We all face challenges in life, and we all have a choice to do something or nothing. Dick Burns chose to do something, and by sharing his experience, he sets the stage for others to follow and help restore the dignity so deserved by stroke survivors.

Jim Baranski
Chief Executive Officer
National Stroke Association

INTRODUCTIONS

The book is written for you. Because you have been given a special gift. You've been given a second chance. Who am I? No one special, but I died and came back to life. So what I've got to say is special.

This is a story about a stroke – the leading cause of long-term disability in the country and the third leading cause of death. On the average, a stroke strikes someone every forty-five seconds. That's about 800,000 people a year. And stroke is becoming more commonplace every day.

This is a story about hope. It is a road map to recovery, what's involved and what's necessary for that recovery, how to come out of it as a whole person and a better person. It tells of personal growth and the resulting satisfaction of a return to life as a functioning, contributing member of society. Nothing is hopeless. You can work miracles – if you know how.

This is a story that can serve as a motivating guide for recovery and treats a fascinating and perplexing subject with the total attention it deserves. It's a factual tale of practical experience that identifies the problems, tells what's involved, what to expect, and how to solve them.. It's about how to cope and conquer how to come out on top and how to live a real life. It's a story that takes a while to play out and challenges some widely held medical dogma along the way. It's a story about the psychological and emotional traumas of battling illness or injury where problems and opportunities can be the same. And, it's a story for any health crisis.

This story is not exactly a memoir, although it is filled with personal history. Nor is it a textbook – even though some parts may seem almost clinical. What it is is a book about choices and directions and hope. It's about being abruptly taken from a familiar life, being battered about, rejected, experiencing powerful emotions, learning how to fight for life and live, and learning about life and people.

This is a story of survival. It's a tale to inform and help. And it's to this fortunate "you" that this book is directed.

Medical science has come a long way, contributing astounding advances. With breathtaking new vistas of biomedicine, there are new strides being taken toward understanding the body and the brain. With regard to the brain, the first and most astounding is called Neurogenesis. For years, medical dogma has held that brain cells, once dead are gone forever. Other parts of the brain may take over functions but it's never enough. But medicine only used the first part of this "theory." The second part essentially said that it was up to scientists and research of the future to prove this "diagnosis" wrong. Well, they have. The same would apply to the great strides made in heart surgery and care and in cancer knowledge and increased survival. And, with other diseases, control and correction.

But, the area that science and medicine cannot fully diagnose and treat is that of the emotions, the personal actions and reactions that impact on function and progress on the path to wellness. Yes, there are guidelines and direction. But the individual challenges remain: how you react to an illness or operation, the demands on body and mind, and just how you deal with them to effect a recovery. Simply: you're sick, medicine, therapy, exercise and regimen, can help make your body well – what does it take to make your mind, your being, your life, well? There's no free lunch. You've got to do this yourself. Medicine calls this Neurogenesis. This book calls it "how."

Some experiences and remembrances offered will be humorous, others sad, some glorious, some unconscionable, some maybe boring. But all are necessary. Relish the moments of laughter because laughter is an essential element to recovery. The ability to laugh at life, particularly at yourself, brings with it ultimate triumph and the ability to rise above the small stuff.

Combined, these chapters tell a tale that can answer many questions, give a new perspective and make a positive difference. Consider it as wisdom from a survivor who went through what you or your loved one has or may be going through now. And my wish is that you find things in this story that will make a positive difference in your life. It's a story for you. To get well, recover and be the best you can be.

CHAPTER ONE

"Say It With Flowers"
(FTD Florists, 1917)

I died that night.

I was abruptly taken from the life I knew by a Cerebral Hemorrhage, or in today's medical terminology, a Hemorrhagic Stroke. The medical staff at the hospital threw up their hands: "Make him comfortable, the body's paralyzed, there's blood all over and the brain's gone. There's nothing we can do." Common knowledge of the time said that that was it, and my wife was advised to make the arrangements, including this article for the newspaper:

OBITUARY NOTICE
December 26, 1968

RICHARD (DICK) BURNS, 38, television and advertising executive who dressed grown men as fruit for an underwear commercial, had an airline paint smiles on their planes, and brought those same smiles to millions of children around the world, died suddenly the day after Christmas. He is survived by his wife, Nancy and three children, Lisa, Shelley and Richard.

Hold on a minute: is this all I have accomplished during my time on this planet? I must have something better to offer than some silly TV ads.

And I guess the Almighty agreed because I didn't die.

The next morning arrived and so did I. I'm not crippled. I'm not mentally retarded (though there are times when I wonder a bit about both.) I have assumed a place in the sun, albeit somewhat reordered from my previous life, seeing the light, accomplishing something for someone besides myself, recognizing the needs and wants of others, helping my fellow man, trying to make my presence really mean something of merit, putting my years of experience to work.

I had to live — and live a life.

CHAPTER TWO

"It Takes A Licking And Keeps On Ticking"
(Timex Watches, 1956)

I lay on a white bed, in a white "gown," in a white cubicle. I stretched a pasty-white and very spare form awkwardly and without too much pain. I looked around. Everything was out of focus — objects, people — just a blur. In puzzlement, I ran a shaking hand through a mass of unkempt brown hair, then across a lined and rather ample forehead.

I'm alive, I thought. *But where am I? And what am I doing here — wherever "here" is?*

Continuing this personal examination, I rubbed a somewhat angular nose, opened a very acrid mouth and the ran my tongue over full and bow-shaped but stiff and dry lips, brought that shaking hand up to feel a whisker-scruffy chin and jut that object out in subconscious defiance.

It was a change from the blackness that had enveloped me, and that long dark abyss that I seemed to have experienced. I looked down at the sparse coverings and thought to myself: *they say that the good guys are always in white and* look at me — *I'm all in white, my body, the cover so I guess I'm one of the good guys. I'm certainly a lucky good guy. Guess I'm not dead because I can more or less move my extremities. Yes, they're all there. Thanks. Whoever. Whatever.*

The mind? I guess that functions. There seemed to be thoughts, rather muddled...not right, not like it used to be. Am I me? Where do I go from here? What will I do? What CAN I do? There's got to be more than just being here. Can I function, can I do, can I?

These and other thoughts rushed through my head.

I tried to look around, as much as I could and tried to get my bearings. I thought, *if the mind works — some, maybe the senses would— some?*

The first thing that hit me was the smell. It was foreign and peculiarly clean, rather like a garage sprayed with perfumed kerosene. Then as I grew used to it, I begin to separate those many smells. There was this antiseptic smell, the dry and powdery smell of pills, the aroma of a multitude of medicines and disinfectants – together with the strong smell of sweat from anxious patients, tempered by the scrubbed soap and water purification of the doctors and nurses as they scurried by my stall.

The second item on my "trying to understand where I was" journey was the sounds. There was constant chatter from the other spaces called "cubicles." Mindless attempts at communication by scared hospital residents and the attempts to sooth and reassure by relations and other visitors. And the voices of the caregivers, also so calming and placating.

There were the sights. Blurry at first. I began to focus on the décor of my space — and it was minimal. A fluorescent light hovered over the bed, which had racks on the sides with buttons and controls. A phone and a button to call for help seemed to sum up the situation. At least I shouldn't feel abandoned. Gauges, tubes, plugs, thermometer-like things, curtains to protect privacy, a closet and chest of drawers and a chair rounded out the scenery. Simply, the space was small and confining. Beyond there were lights, larger spaces, more lights, more rooms. Everything looked the same in the nothingness of the artificial light.

As is common in places of illness and recuperation, there were lanes of people hustling to and fro. Nurses breezed by in their starched gowns; doctors made their rounds, checking vital signs, listening, then making notes on those charts hung precariously on the ends of the beds, other people came and went – volunteers and orderlies cleaning, emptying, banging mops and containers. I watched, and helplessly tried to speak to them, question them. But I guess my efforts were but noises, mixed with those other groans and sighs constantly emanating from my helpless companions. They were sounds to be ignored in favor of business, the business of this place.

A concerned-looking and seemingly attentive nurse stepped up to my side with an inquisitive look. And the wheels that were my brain ("once and future" - as it's said) began to turn. Maybe she'll help, tell me where, what. I opened my mouth to communicate, cry out for answers. Dry lips parted, a mealy tongue moved.

Only guttural and primal-sounding noises came out.

I'm just out of practice, I hoped. Rationalizing, I tried again.

More guttural and primal sounds.

Oh, Lord. Help me!

The reality of what might be overwhelmed me and that watery stuff began to spill out the sides of my normally calm and focused brown eyes.

I was now reduced to sniveling misery. *Good thing no one can see me, bad for the image and all that.* Then I thought to myself: *Oh, who in the hell really cares.* My thoughts wandered aimlessly...

Then, after a while, as a harbinger of things to come into my life, into that very muddled state of mind came some very clear and meaningful thoughts: (a "destroyed" brain and "meaningful" thoughts meant there had to be an inner voice or a dream or something else doing the talking)...

There comes a time in life when you have to take a stand, no matter the dangers, no matter the what. This is that time. Oh, yeah, there'll be ups and downs. But, just maybe I can come out of all this, make a difference, accomplish good things. This is an opportunity. This is my challenge! I'm alive, not dead. I can move my limbs. I must still have more or less a mind, even though I can't communicate...I think I can function...I will function.

Yes. Take a step. Forward. One at a time. It may take a while. Yes, I will do it!

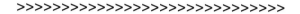

But the effort must have been too much. The eyelids gently shut down; the sounds around me gradually silenced, and my mind slipped into the past. I started to dream, I guess, reminiscing and reflecting about what must have brought me to this point.

CHAPTER THREE
"Come To Where The Flavor Is"
(Philip Morris & Co., Inc., 1967)

New York City beckoned, and I had jumped at the chance because this was the center of my chosen world.

Those overpowering structures of steel, glass and mortar that lined the avenues of Manhattan are at once an imposing sight and a man-made fortification designed to keep the rigors of nature at bay. They seemed to symbolize much of what this country is about ,that which is this country, structures of ego and undeniable achievement reaching to the heavens to entreat support and sustain our way of life. As I thought so many times much later, there was little doubt as to why those suicidal terrorists chose New York and Manhattan skyscrapers as their target.

For many reasons, including ability, luck and the challenge of it all, I had begun my business life in that fledgling entertainment medium called television. And, New York was the business center. Fast becoming a fashionable tool to reflect the values of a new and quickening lifestyle, this medium was informing and influencing life — and I was on top and felt like showing off a little. Oh, the impetuousness and naiveté of youth and its flawed perception of life. I guess I was a pretty fair "Man in the Gray Flannel Suit" as people in my business were known in those days. Whatever physical prowess possessed was hidden behind tailored natural-shoulder, three-piece suits and dark glasses that made for a studious yet adventurous appearance. Sunglasses regardless of the weather or time were the rage, looking mysterious while making thoughts unreadable, the person, unfathomable. Most in my world thought that I had done well for one so young, for still in my early thirties I'd been chosen to lead a part of a large national conglomerate in an aggressive new sales endeavor. I was excited. I was honored. I was stimulated by the challenge. I was in a state of awe. But I wasn't humbled.

Yet.

A business giant offered this particular challenge. It was the Philadelphia-Reading Corporation, composed of successful companies and successful people. These individual companies were giants in themselves: the railroad of the same name, steel, boots, clothing, and that new operation (mine?) that the skeptics questioned and gave little hope — toys. Remember the big ones, Topper toys that were sold in the supermarkets, stacked above you while you were shopping (that was a key distribution factor) and advertised continuously on children's television shows around the country? Topper Toys even had its own show. Remember "Rocky and Bullwinkle." And I can remember lots of products, but one stands out — the doll.

My friend, Louis Armstrong, was doing the commercial with those young girls dancing and singing and the pretty little doll, Suzy Cute, that it was all about. The doll, with the arms and legs that moved on command. But, Louie couldn't get it right — instead of "you push her tummy and her arms go up" he kept saying: "you push her tummy and she throws up..." Oh, a special experience. Five takes and then a "jam" session to ease the pain.

I remember Secret Sam, Johnny Seven and Johnny Eagle and Johnny Express, Multi-pistol and Crimebuster with all the scopes and silencers, rocket and grenade launchers to match those of the "bad guys." And there was Baby Boo, Penny Brite, Baby Brite, with the clothes and furniture and dishes to match - all the cars and guns, all the stuff that little girls and boys used to play with and fantasize their drama of growing-up.

It took about nine months to gestate this new operation and make a workable sales and promotional program, develop a saleable and viable product with the packaging to display it and the promotion to reach the people. Almost overnight, a new success. But success always has a price.

Life wasn't all work and no play. There were gourmet events, parties, opera, symphony, theater, museums, galleries, the buildings, the parks, the opulence and the crudeness, and the basics of life. And the people: the young, the old, the in-between, the strivers, the sedate, the complacent, the social and the "hope to be's" and the "doers and the doees".

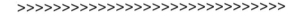

Two incidents stand out as particularly descriptive of our unique way of life in this new, faster-paced, productive world — and what was waiting around the corner. In retrospect, I think I can realistically say that these differences and, similarities, are what make this country, and us, strong. The people are diverse, from different backgrounds and ways of this world and life, creative and visionary, individually and collectively. Put it all together and you've got winners

That's what this story is all about.

The first example was a social affair — a formal dinner at our house, The guests were a select group of neighborhood and business friends. We were a very fortunate, All-American family. I had a good job with good pay so that we could afford a good life and a domicile that we called a house (the home would come later.) I can see the place, the setting, even now, years later … the house that showed off by itself. Set back from paved world by a sculptured lawn, nestled in the green of pine and birch. It was a traditional white of generous wood construction with a long walkway through a greenery of lawns and trees that ended at an inset door   That door that opened to an imposing entry that led to living room of passable size and decoration and sizeable seating ability. Then the long dining room with it's high ceilings, perfect for entertaining, beckoned guests. Outside from a relaxing den-room, we had attempted to fashion a Japanese-style garden out of the landscaping - to the dismay of our conservative neighbors (yet, what could be more orderly and conservative than mathematical groupings of rock, streams and bushes) - oriental tranquility and symmetry was very popular in the West but so different and seemly awkward in the East.

Our recently acquired and fashionable friends, in a dilemma as to the appropriate attire, bent their collective heads together and decided that people from the West were really still "savages" and so this affair was probably nothing more than a fancy barbecue. I can't help but chuckle, recalling their mortification upon being greeted by my wife, in a long, flowing gown and a host in black tie, whilst they, in Bermuda shorts, showing off knobby knees, were accompanied by ladies with light and airy fashionable dresses and other vacation attire. Their collective "faux pas" left them awkward and speechless. Was this just a flawed perception of our life, or was this a way of testing us, training us in anticipation of what was to come?

The second occasion was a unique gathering of the advertising heads of the corporate divisions of the firm. It started out as a "let's meet for drinks" gathering and it became the genesis of one of the country's best-known and successful advertising efforts. The scene was a well-known watering hole and bistro in Manhattan's Plaza Hotel, called the "Oak Room." And the cast was six grown business executives, intelligent and soon-to-be creative souls. The room was dark, decorated with compatible hand-hewn black oak tables and chairs, wood paneled walls with paintings of grand people looking down with gentle smiles as if knowing what was to happen.

One of the divisions of the company was having difficulty in communicating the need and usefulness of its product to consumers. Especially with pictures and the new medium of television. For the` problem was the product: men's cotton underwear. Making underwear socially acceptable and moving millions to buy was the challenge. So, how to effectively communicate and motivate?

The evening reflected camaraderie, much wassail and drinking and some good old-fashioned marketing smarts. And then, creatively, the Division's dilemma was resolved and the unique "Fruit Of The Loom" advertising campaign was born.

"Yes, you should be the banana," and we so annointed the tall, spare advertising V.P. of one division. He reminded us all of a vaudevillian "Top Banana." And, "you can handle being a pear rather well," we generously appointed another who was robust and round with bottom to match. "A fig for you!" as we assigned another stalwart and the remaining "awards" were hilariously offered by a chorus of voices, "And an orange and a lemon."

"And an apple a day keeps everyone imbibing," slurred another.

To get even, the new banana offered: "This is a bar, isn't it? So let's not forget the grape." And so by unanimous agreement, I became the grape, soon to be crushed, later to be remolded into a fine wine.

Imagine the scene. Six vested (coats were off by now) grown men, powerful executives, imitating the being of six quasi-human, fruity characters. The words, the actions, the emotions, the hilarity — this was the beginning of what was to become a television classic. It was so simple: humor would always captivate — and sell. Each "fruit" would come alive, portrayed as a person, becoming a part of the need, the appeal of the product, dramatizing each piece of the sales puzzle. And it was as much fun to devise as it must have been for those lucky souls later developing the concept and the marketing success that followed. The logo and commercials may differ a bit, but they didn't have six divisions and six very happy, high-powered egos to consider.

The point is clear: however important, influential or powerful, we must remind ourselves that we are all equal in the ability to be productive and effective. How productive, how effective is how we deal with the hand we are dealt.

CHAPTER FOUR
"The Antidote For Civilization"
(Club Med, 1982)

The job in the East was done. The West was calling. The first act had ended and a second and new act had begun. A new adventure loomed. I had found that life was pretty much like playing a violin solo in public and learning the instrument as I went along. This homily was soon to prove so important.

The children were sent west by air while the furniture explored the country by van. My wife and I meandered through history and geography across this land. We were guided by my wife's Eastern background and our interests, places which, heretofore, I had only read about. I found that those tall tales were mostly true. We experienced New England at the beautiful and colorful turning of the leaves. We explored, found parts of our heritage in old villages and streets and the people and buildings and antique shops. We relived the struggles, the battles, the colors, the growing pains of our young nation and the sounds of those years past — the beat of marching feet, the rattle of drums, the piercing sound of pipes, even heard the tranquility and anguish of our native people. This was Northeast America and this was Canada where culture and history is so similar and we found that here is where it all started. This is where early America lived and fought and learned aand took it's first steps — the French and Indian Wars, then the Revolutionary War, the Congress, the Constitution. What a history lesson.

Exploring more across this land, we found the vast productivity of our heartland, the beauty and squalor of our cities, the jagged earth and rock of millenniums of nature's changes, some parts blanketed with snow and bathed in a deep blue sky overhead. The vast expanses of the arid calm of the desert fascinated us. Finally those silent, rolling golden-brown hills dotted with hues of green scrub and oak and the black shapes of grazing animals welcomed us. We were home, and life was good.

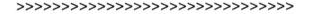

We paid a visit to our new home on the eastern side of San Francisco Bay — space and possibilities ready to challenge an ambitious twosome, Colonial style with silent dormers overlooking a quiet street and a lake. Picture postcard. And I thought: *Could the world be any better?* But those silent and stoic dormers looked out at something unknown — my wife and the house saw something that I didn't, or wouldn't or couldn't. Because, she abruptly collapsed down on the floor and unreasonably wept. As if on cue, it began to rain and streams of water also began to run down the face of those dormers. They were trying to tell me something. Why couldn't I hear?

Why couldn't I see a life soon to be shattered?

The house was appropriately in a bedroom community across the Bridge from that Baghdad by the Bay called San Francisco. While we were in New York, the area had changed, grown with many new developments and citizens. But, "the City" (as affectionately called) hadn't changed that much. It was still the sophisticated-appearing, internationally-melded and oft provincial city I remembered. I compared it now to that which I had left, for the sun shown brightly throughout the day on an easier-going populace — no skyscrapers here, just buildings and a more relaxed people and slower-moving way of life.

The adrenaline flowed to meet the challenges of building a new business. Advertising. My partners and I felt the best way to serve our economy (and make a buck while maximizing limited staff capability) was to concentrate on smaller, local businesses that needed the right direction. Business came and business went, people came and people went. There were the clients, of both sexes, loud and boisterous, timid and quiet, but often with a big carrot for the world, new ideas and new ways for a new and different life.

It was exciting, yet tenuous, for life was sweet and satisfying but underneath it all ran that current that said this wasn't the answer. That so-easy solution to all seemed a merger with a larger and established business. Oh, I remember them clearly. They shall remain anonymous so as to protect the guilty (explanations later.) There was the large, often short-sighted one with the sharp features, sharper tongue and the track record of being a "hard type." There was the handsome front man who lived off creative successes of the past. There was the blasé, younger gigolo with the sharp mind and an astoundingly continuous creative ability. And, as all the stories portray, there was the pencil-faced, "Yes-Man," who covered all the others' mistakes — legally. But I innocently and stupidly ignored the obvious and convinced myself that it was just the right fit. I also convinced myself that the environment would be stimulating and that I could certainly handle any problems with a staff of people to support and augment my efforts, my needs. Creative juices to make the economic world bear fruit had already begun to flow. Ego had taken charge. It felt right and it was so easy. I couldn't see then that I was so steadily slipping into a hedonistic and unrealistic life.

But, that didn't matter. Yet.

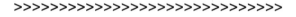

My most un-favorite night nurse barged into this reverie and in a wet, limpid tone said, "How are we tonight? Roll over, it's time for our shots."

How much time for me — I wondered?

CHAPTER FIVE
"You Can Trust Your Car To The Man Who Wears The Star"
(Texaco, 1961)

Was it morning? I had pretty much lost track of time. The weather hadn't. It was funky and foggy. As dull a day outside as it was in. Even the curtains hung loosely around our beds. Why, I wondered, did no one in here seem to function or even care? *Good morning, Mr. Negative.*

Fortunately, the good doctor was there. Cy was our family doctor and a good friend, professionally and socially. He was stout, jovial, outgoing and a gentleman. Belying this jovial appearance, his face shouted strength of character, knowledge and experience. A balding head and firm mouth told anyone who took the trouble to hear that he was the sovereign of one's health and recovery. Yet there was that dimpled chin and crow's feet that signaled humor. He was a wise one. His advice and encouragement had helped this patient through both good and bad times.

When the stroke hit me, he abruptly left a full waiting room of patients to temporarily fend for themselves while he contained a crisis. Such is the value of friendship. It was only later that I learned that he was medical and administrative head of the hospital to which he directed my paramedic saviors. Small wonder actions were so swift.

"You certainly gave us all a few fits and starts, my friend," he proclaimed, laying a cold stethoscope's mouth on my forehead, then my chest, listening for telltale sounds.

"How much do you remember after you blacked out? You've been in a deep coma yesterday and last night, but now it seems that you've decided to come back to us. The Hospital called Nancy and told her that she'd better make the arrangements. Shirley (Cy's wife) went to be with her, hold her hand and all. Then, Nancy's turn to call me this morning saying that everyone was flabbergasted, the paralysis had passed, you were looking better and she figured that you'd fight through whatever. We knew then that you had come back to us. Can you talk? Can you communicate at all?"

I looked up from my prone position and slurred a response, hoping that Cy could understand, (guess it was more or less coherent) — "Guess I gave you all some bad times, I'm so sorry, but I think I know why this all happened and it's going to work out OK..." I mouthed this with simulated.

Conviction and then my voice faltered (gee, I could talk some or at least communicate. There was hope?)

Cy persisted and verbally probed: "OK, you'd had the eye surgery and everything seemed fine. Let's figure out what you did, or didn't do, that made all this happen."

Eye surgery had started the whole mess. It was necessitated by broken glasses at a 1967

Super Bowl party and the subsequent disclosure of a detached retina. The operation that followed required drastically turning the eye around, which obviously triggered the calamitous result. I returned home from the hospital and surgery with bandaged eyes, no hurt, just inconvenience, existing like a deprived being, eating by positioning food items and placing utensils like the face of a clock, and hearing, not seeing and blissfully sleeping to relieve the humdrum boredom. It was Christmas time, vacation for the children, work for my wife, drudgery for me. Little did I know what was next on the agenda in a few short weeks.

I thought some about all this and then attempted a reply, somewhat slurred, haltingly and somewhat coherently, and the essence was: "I guess we don't always know what's in us, because I didn't do anything that wasn't prescribed by you and the eye guy. I took the medicines, I ate what I was supposed to, the way I was supposed to, I rested, but it all just happened anyway."

Cy continued, "Like a heart attack. A shock, if you will. Like a seizure. Some call it apoplexy. Simply, you had a stroke. A Cerebral Hemorrhage to be exact, medically speaking, an Arterial Fistula. An artery burst in the back of your head, flooding the whole cranial cavity, systematically destroying your brain cells — top to bottom. You were brain dead. Anyone in your family have this kind of problem?"

"Don't know," I muttered, struggling to respond. "No one ever lived long enough to tell me."

There is so much still to learn about medicine, about ourselves. Life is a mixture of both good and bad and one has to look at it for the long haul – and create a balance.

Just then there was a commotion up front in the Intensive Care Unit (ICU) Raised voices swept down the Ward. .Especially one with a solicitous, yet firm voice of authority.

"I'm his wife, and I'm a friend and patient of the doctor. I am going in to see my husband and I really don't give a 'fig' for whatever rules you have made up." (In those days, visitors were not welcome in the ICU.)

"Please move out of the way. Thank you." And with that, a lovely vision blew into the ward. She was a petite blond lady with hair purposely casual, artfully concealing a clear, intelligence-reeking forehead and knowing, sparkling eyes peering out from a visage of clear, flushed complexion. Her firm jaw was set, proclaiming determination and character and a "don't tread on me" look that said the beauty was more than skin-deep.

She came to a stop beside my cubicle. She brushed the good Doctor's cheek and bent over me, throwing her strong arms about my frail body and planted a gentle but firm kiss. Nancy, my wife, my friend, my partner in life, had arrived.

"Welcome back to me, us, the world. You had us all so terrified. Please don't give us any more problems, Love. Thank God for you - from the children, from me, from all of us. What's the story, Cy, how is he, how long, when can he come home, when, how..." heart-shaped lips trembled a bit, her voice a bit high and she held onto her only 38-year-old husband a little tighter as it must have been rather hard keeping a "stiff upper lip" with all the emotion just waiting to be released.

Sensing the moment's pressure, Cy calmly interjected the medical verdict: "Oh, probably about another one or two weeks in here and then another two-three weeks in the main hospital. Then other hospitals for testing and special care. You'll just have to work around this whole thing, my dear. He's a very sick man. His brain and his body are wasted and destroyed. It'll be a long while before he's ready to resume anything like his former life and for some things, never. Forget about sports, no more singing, no piano, things that he did before – anything that requires coordination. But he'll think, move, breathe, do, and eventually lead a fairly normal life."

A bleak prognosis for the future.
The world had just come down on my head. And it hurt!.
Where do we go from here? And, if it's that bad - how?

CHAPTER SIX
"It Puts Off Old Age"
(Quaker Oats Cereals, 1902)

Hospital life is what you make it, a grateful rest from the rigors of every day or just a dreary and boring existence. Well, I couldn't make anything, so it was just that — schedules, discipline and order with no obvious rewards. Or so it seemed.

The routines are set as the best way to get a patient better in preparation for re-entering life. I tried to view everything, the hospital and the routines, as a temporary prison of health. Any small glimpse of eventual freedom and wellness was a victory to be celebrated.

The next month, spent under the close scrutiny of the busy nurses and specialists of Intensive Care, I was a problem. Anyone subjected to a debilitating illness like a heart attack, a cancer, an arterial or venial issue, a serious injury, needs to understand that there's going to be a change in personality and demeanor. When the body has been ravished and devastated, bombarded with medicines and drugs and the brain needs to cope with the trauma, the patient most commonly will experience "mental irregularities," differences in behavior. Which is a polite way of saying, "freaks out."

My behavior became the opposite of what it

had been.   Before the stroke I was rather neat and ordered, proud and restrained. Now, my actions became undisciplined and, obviously revolting against hospital rules and restraints, I shouted obscenities at the slightest provocation and proceeded to throw bedpans and urine bags at the unsuspecting staff.   Easily frightened, I was duly restrained by a full component of male nurses and orderlies (adversity gives one added physical strength.) I freed myself of such things as intravenous feeding tubes, and instead, sticking same into the mattress that seemingly needed it more than I, pulled out a catheter because it was uncomfortable, even escaped from a straight jacket. Stupidly proud and unjustified.

I would take medicines and laxatives only after being tricked into believing that they were vintage wines. Then there was the incident of directing the entire ward of bedridden patients to walk to salvation. I can see that ludicrous picture, like the march from Prokofiev's "The Love of Three Oranges" where an entire cast of servants and principals (here, patients, nurses and doctors) marched in protest to nonsense.

Small wonder they tested me for psychiatric aberrations.   The truth is that illness is accompanied by misery, self-indulgence with a short fuse. One wants the rest of the world to feel just as miserable. Child like tantrums are just a way to avoid facing the truth.

But how about the hospital staff, those selfless people who were trying to help me while I was making their jobs hard? There were many, but let me call attention to two specific nurses, with contrasting looks and behavior, that contributed greatly to my recovery. First let's describe a day nurse. She was responsible for the daytime tedium. (And that was herself.) On the outside she was all woman, a beautiful creature of statuesque proportions disguised in a starched, white and scary dress. This was Glenda, and although she looked like that good witch from the "Wizard of Oz," her attitude and actions belied the appearance as she acted more like Adelpha, the Wicked Witch of the West, riding her broom to our doom. We covertly named her "Miss Efficiency" (and other names behind her back).

Her job was to succor the poor unfortunates who made up the "ICKY" (as the Intensive Care Unit was affectionately called), and she did it with such aloofness and disregard of facts and need as to wither the hopes of the most optimistic of patients.

Miss Efficiency would regularly sweep into the wards, the cubicles, and pronounce to all: "Today I want to make sure that each of you is properly shaved and bathed in order that you are presentable to the important people who are coming to visit you. Also, each of you will remain composed and appear comfortable at all times. Remember, we're all happy to be here and be sure to say that you all just love what I do for you. We're all in this together and I want you to show gratitude." And the nurses aids and other hospital flunkies descended upon us and scrubbed, moved, scraped, smoothed, fluffed and redid our bodies and surroundings so that all glittered and glistened. And, I mused: *newly shorn and dressed lambs to the slaughter…*

This activity was a weekly routine. The rest of the time we mostly floundered on our own. I seem to remember a time when I was left unattended, naked and unshaven, shivering in cold mute misery.

But all was not lost. A shift in our fortunes brought the opportunity of a lovely angel of mercy. We were saved. A new nurse.

Let's call her "Nurse Happiness." She was plain to look at but animated and open in her demeanor and actions, married with children of her own. Starched gown was something that disguised some physical short-comings but it was her face that gave her away. The features were strong and the tender, dancing eyes, the laughing mouth told of her willing involvement with life. And her hair, the crown of her being, was so lovely and glossy as to seemingly hold a perpetual halo above it. She knew her business and she knew about life, and she cared. And she gave. This was Florence Nightingale reborn, for she brought happiness to our otherwise "humdrum" existence. We looked forward to her presence. And we responded accordingly. Her habit was to visit each of us individually, ask with interest about our well-being (or lack thereof), our wants and needs, our lives. She would stimulate our sense of being and coerce us to accept and move beyond our problems. The melodious voice interestingly inquired about our progress and knowingly found out what the doctors needed to learn about each patient's progress. That chart at the bottom of the bed told the overt statistical and physical story but "Nurse Happiness" could divine the real progress, tell the real story.

And, the real story was that we all made progress, minute at times, but enough to eventually get me out of that place into the hospital proper.

And, my adventures were just starting.

CHAPTER SEVEN
"The Great Escape"
(Bavarian Motor Works, 1973)

To set the stage: the weather outside was damp and grey with little breaks as the sun tried to peek through the overcast and into the starved hearts of we poor creatures huddled under the bedclothes inside. At this juncture we remained warm and secure in our semi-conscious state, determining that the real world out there was just too dangerous. Cy came to visit early this day. It had been decided that special testing was in order and that other hospitable venues were needed:

"Gather your strength, my friend, you're going on a trip. The hospital will transfer your few belongings and you are moving!"

To what turned out to be the first of three hospitals, those "new" hospitals Cy had spoken of earlier, each with its own specialties of testing and repair.

They whisked me by rooms with swinging doors, down a maze of hallways with lights peering at me from above, by staircases that must go somewhere, wheeled me onward – floors, elevators and rapidly moving people flashed by my vision. Until the fresh wind of life quenched my breath. I was outside. This is good, I thought. I wasn't so afraid any longer.

In fact, I wanted to stay out. Oh, for a moment longer. Not to be. I was raised on the gurney and pushed into the back of that portable hospital called an ambulance. Off we went. I tried to keep my eyes open but they must have given me something, because the lids got soooooo heavyyyyyy...

The motion stopped. I was there. Wherever. A repeat of the past performance, in reverse, as I was wheeled out the back of the ambulance, that mobile hospital, through the hallways, through the elevator, down the corridors, into a new and lighter and airier place. Why was it so nice? I thought, was what was to come so bad?

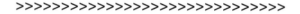

Hospital One was a grand old establishment, an imposing building from a past era. Long drive up to a Mediterranean-style balustrade, ever so reminiscent of those grand hotels of that past. Behind massive stucco walls under the expanse of a tile roof was a large, dark, reception area with too comfortable, over stuffed furniture, fashionable pictures and art-deco fixtures.

As I was soon to learn, I was here for basic body tests.

The next days were spent drifting in and out of a battery of those tests: needles in the arms, little spot bandages on the body and the head, wires and machines monitoring and taking pictures. I learned later that the tests were the same. Only the doctors and specialists who interpreted were the difference.

"Sit-up." "Lie down." "Roll over." "Give me this arm." "Does this hurt?" I really couldn't tell much as I was floating above it all. Procedures were sometimes very painful as medical science wasn't nearly as advanced as it is today. Drawing blood was an experience. Being hooked-up to an Intravenous drip was a happening. There were needles of various sizes, under the skin, on the hand, the wrist, the arm, "no sound, please," and see if the "white coat syndrome" hadn't affected the reading. (Anticipation of the worst when you see a doctor and the blood pressure goes up in anticipation – but why should I be concerned, I couldn't think much at all.) But the best was yet to come. "Make a fist.and pop out that vein." *"Ouch"* when the needle pierced my body.

And they pulled out so much blood I thought I'd turn white from anemia. "Takes about an hour to analyze," they mumbled, "Yes, that other test will have to wait."

All this to find out what? That with time things might turn out mostly right. For whom? Them? My problem was simpler: how much time and how much right?

The food was rather good. But the nerves controlling the muscles needed to swallow and digest were not. The food track and assimilation process had been paralyzed, so I had to learn how to swallow and eat all over again. (Later, I learned that due to Vagas nerve damage, an esophageal stricture had partially closed the passage into the stomach, eventually causing a hernia and an acid reflux problem and ulcers.) Who said life was easy? Chew well and good luck.

It was also in this hospital that the white-coated phantom presence (Or so it seemed to me) of a psychiatrist visited. I seemed to know his game right away, called him a "shrink." To make a long story short, he couldn't understand why the brain was still working after what had happened. He noted that I reacted, slowly, but effectively, and that I seemed to be able to more or less think.

He recommended further testing.

Hurray ! Someone was on my side!

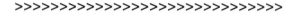

Hospital Two was another factory of medical science. But, unlike Hospital One, Hospital Two was efficiency-oriented, with square-like buildings and décor, sprawling without a pattern, across many city blocks. It was all functional, with flat roofs and swinging doors in front that must have countless stories to tell about tragedies, recovery and relief. These roofs covered bleak but efficient look-alike rooms, dressed in cold and sterile ambience. The beds were obviously to be used for housing as many people in as short a time as possible. This was a cold place that spawned a cold attitude.

Here, they tried to read my mind, find out what made me "tick," find out what to do next. An operation? For what purpose? (they couldn't do much in those days.) Why take the chance? (Now, they can do miracles with rewiring and redoing the damaged body.)

They ran a series of more sophisticated

tests, with more sophisticated equipment.

Use it or lose it, as the saying goes.

First was an EKG, and I couldn't figure out why the "alphabet soup" name because all they did was put little plastic connectors on my body and then hooked up wires to a computer machine with big rolls of paper on wheels and pins on the ends of thick wires that spit out pages with hen scratches all over. I wondered: *hope someone can make more sense of all this than I.*

But this test was a piece of cake

The second test was very painful.

It was an angiogram. Similar to the first, but with wires and things to the head, dye into the blood, and the head placed on a TV-like, X-ray screen that took pictures while I suffered electric pulses that hurt like hell. (I had an occasion to have this test recently and there was no pain at all — thank you, modern science.)

The third was a special one consisting of different kinds of breathing and activity, exertion tests. (Today they do it with machines that take pictures and register capacity and capability. They call it a "Stress Test.") It was interesting when there's no balance to maintain body and foot coordination on a treadmill.

Last, they tried a biopsy. How does one do a biopsy on one's head? In my case, testing a piece of nothing from a nothing — my brain? But I guess they knew what they needed, were doing. (They had hope, too.) Today, they roll you into a big photo-copier with circles of cameras and things that roll around you as you are inside and take pictures of everything about you and pull out any needed tissue with a special needle.

Then, same procedure, much more primitive and it, too, hurt. With today's modern tests, there's no pain at all.

Medicine's specialists abounded here and the nurses ran in and out of my life. There was one doctor who stands out in my memory. Without him, the motivation to survive might have flown. This was a doctor on loan for special study from a big hospital in the East. I became his main study. He was a cold one, all business, no humor. My continued existence astounded him. Perplexed by my progress and confused by the continuing symptoms, he told me later that medicine hadn't progressed enough yet for doctors and specialists to have the necessary medical case studies and information to understand what had happened and what would be the best type of treatment.

And my job was to be one of those case studies.

"Can you hear me?" he would always ask. And since my replies were mostly unintelligible, he would turn to the nurse for assurance and a hopefully coherent collaboration.

"Yes, Doctor," they would always reply, "He's still with us today. And what tests do you want?"

He'd read the chart and thoughtfully comment (more to himself), "This one needs an Angiogram (or whatever). Maybe we can find something that makes him work. Maybe we can open him up and see for ourselves."

All this as if I weren't there.

In my semi-functioning state of mind I knew then that I had to fight through whatever so that

I could show them all, what was wrong, what I was made of and how it could be made right.

No "opening up" *my head. No, not for me*!

And they didn't operate. Thanks to my wife. Gambles with life didn't always work back then. The odds are almost a sure thing today.

But then we're getting ahead of the story.

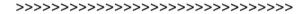

Hospital Three was my next stop. It was referred to as the "Country Club" of hospitals (why not, they served wine with dinner, a very unusual "plus" in those days). It was a modern structure, recently built. It was set in a bustling city area away from other medical establishments. It was one story, square, of modern architecture, with plain walls and plain roofs, with windows that really opened. Windows that looked out on green trees and shrubbery that shouted tranquility in the midst of the hurried business of life.

But this outside disguised the inside of efficiency and professional ambience. There was a smallish reception area that opened to a huge expanse of orderly beds, full of people, and seemingly everywhere, a hustling and efficient staff. Here was a professional, yet warm atmosphere of constant attention. Doctors were competent, even better, good.

I remember this hospital well as it was a very special experience.

Here, they were to repair the damage incurred when I ripped out the catheter in that first hospital. The night shift and the doctor on duty, the nurses, never put it back, stopped up my waterworks and made for medical problems that have lasted. The procedure went well (although some small problems remain to remind me of responsibility and the grand rewards of life).

It was repaired to a point where I could more or less function on my own.

My hopes were rewarded, my wishes answered — I could go home!

But, if I could have thought clearly, I would have been frightened: no staff of professionals to help, on my own, alone to begin the fight back. No, not alone: my wife, my children, my friends would rally 'round my bedside.

At last, I could look forward to a future of happiness and hope?

CHAPTER EIGHT
"Don't Leave Home Without It"
(American Express Company, 1975)

They say that home is where the heart is. I took heart because I knew that home is where I could think, hopefully straighter, and figure this whole thing, and me, out.

But home lacked the medical conveniences and trained staff to monitor and help my recovery, so it presented many problems. Years later, I reflected that this was a good thing. Because I had to learn how to solve problems on my own, and I found that solving those many problems myself was the best way to get better and grow up. It was a beneficial trade-off. But at the time it seemed like too much, too soon.

In honor of my homecoming, the day was the first good looking one of many. Before, the weather seemed to always match my mood and the situation — a foggy funk. Now, the sun burned brightly in the blue sky and it matched the mood of happiness, anticipation and hope.

Feelings? Returning home gave me a marvelous sense of freedom, of almost indescribable relief, an overwhelming feeling of security, yet of release from a long guardianship and now the ability (and challenge) to function on my own. And maybe a little fear of what might be.

For convenience my bedroom was moved to the dining room. The prisms of glass on the chandelier overhead were great in the daylight, but, ever try to sleep at night with dancing streams of light, of the moon, stars, cars, brightly dancing off the walls? It's fascinating, yet distracting as it makes for strange Rorschach pictures. (For I could more or less psychoanalyze myself — I thought.)

The bathroom was a challenge. Out of bed, on the floor, struggle upright, only a short way, but leaving handprints most everywhere. Ablutions took about two hours at first, and shaving without serious injury was a chore to be dreaded. (For some inexplicable reason, my skin wouldn't yet tolerate an electric razor.)

There was little remarkable about those first days. Days turned into weeks, weeks to months. Eat, sleep, exercise as the body permitted. Practice speaking so that it doesn't come out mushy and jumbled. The brain knew what I was trying to say but obviously the mouth didn't. There were interesting attempts at navigation, trying valiantly to function when the body doesn't — and can't. Such attempts included crawling, hobbling, lurching and even some "walking" with those fingerprints all over the walls, doors and anything else that I could hold on to. Next was the cane stage. It helped — but not enough. And, it was Nancy who finally had enough. Yanking the cane from me one day as we were outside, "walking" around that beautiful lake (really just a reservoir for watering that country club golf course but I couldn't tell the difference — it was just lovely green-blue water) she broke it and appropriately expounded: "God gave you two legs, use them!" I tried, harder. It began to work.

It certainly was easy to greet people, being close to the door, in the front of the house. They were mostly my wife's friends as mine were scarce. Came to find out later that they were afraid of me, or rather afraid that what had happened to me could happen to them.

Television became a companion. I remember avidly watching the morning news, jousting with quiz show panels, whetting my appetite with culinary adventures, becoming immersed in the trivia and emotionalism of the soaps. Mostly it was mindless company to pass the time. Later, I realized that it made me imagine and think. Therapy? I was mesmerized by that brilliant tube with light and sound and action and was forced to watch all those commercials I had made and sold. Retribution? Being an old broadcaster, I pondered the programming and production, thinking that it could be so much more (better?) for so many. Like the old radio soaps and serials where the imagination ran amuck. And, in those days, television still reflected society, presented that which garnered audiences. It was the good which made us think positively, not the negative or sensational. It didn't try to define or influence, imposing standards or politicizing. I call it "purple journalism." It's a propaganda and numbers game now.

During those tedious days of recovery, there were some important happenings from the very first, things that would forever influence my life and that of my family. And from these occurrences I learned to listen to the advice of those who loved me, who had my best interests at heart, and who cared. To that I added the advice of experience. I melded the two.

Togetherness is not just a phrase on greeting cards. It's a part of what helped me through it all.

CHAPTER NINE
"Look, Ma, No Cavities"
(Crest Toothpaste, 1958)

There were down times, black moments. I thought I'd never recover. Yet, life is like walking, one foot in front of the other, slowly, purposefully, one step at a time and pretty soon I'd reach the goal. Maybe the similes are overworked, but I just reached down deep inside, and pulled myself up by the bootstraps, as they say. Guess I had more guts and moxie than I thought, and finding this strength, I used it.

Well, I thought, (I'm thinking!) at least I have a job. There'll be enough income for this house. Money to put food on the table. A way to support my wife and the children   What I didn't expect were the new challenges that life was going to throw at me.

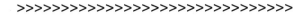

The first warning of the many things that were to happen in my new, struggling existence was the arrival of a letter. Those business associates, presumably partners but obviously unaware of the meaning of obligation and loyalty, decided to "lose" my contract, ignore the agreements. And lose me. My illness presented the opportunity for them to have it all — keep all the monies from the accounts and yet pay out no salary and no benefits and have no one around to keep it all honest. I could think, feel emotion by now because all at once I was surprised, flabbergasted, devastated, and angry. They had assured my wife that all would be fine, not to worry.

This whole matter haunts me even to this day. They bad-mouthed me and blackballed me in business. They fabricated and planted stories so that eventually I had to look outside my profession for gainful employment. As if my physical and mental problems weren't enough of a challenge. Whatever happened to honesty and morality? They only cared about themselves, their "needs."

Fortunately I had a disability insurance policy. Unfortunately, I just hadn't read all the fine print that involved using Social Security and a limitation on payments. How can anyone support a family of five on $1000.00 a month? Especially with me as I was?

Suddenly there was no income. We had some savings but that wouldn't last long Life, such as it was, looked pretty grim.

Then along came the promoters and shady entrepreneurs. They were not only vultures, but also opportunists, with their own interests at heart, certainly not mine. Just work a few days a week at home. You hear it, read it in the media, now on the Internet. Put your experience to work for only a small investment. Make a fortune. Don't worry. Hah! Many are referred to as Pyramid organizations and you might as well go for the lotto because the odds are as good (unless you get in first and out first).

And then there were the old friends who handled the necessary requirements of existence like the attorneys, the bankers, the insurance agents and stockbrokers, They wouldn't listen to Nancy, who vainly tried to tell the way it was with me, because, for sure, I couldn't make any sensible decisions. Guess they all had their own agenda. Everyone was an expert and wanted to give good news. Everyone wanted to "help." Most, for a fee. Draw your own conclusions.

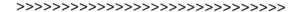

One occurrence cries for detail because it tells the whole story. A former business associate came calling, flattered my ego by offering that which was denied — work. The job was the promotion of a new product line. Like my past successes. I bought into it. After much discussion, mostly argumentative, I was allowed to work with strict boundaries and guidelines for others to watch me and guide me. They did not. Greed got in the way and tragedy was the necessary consequence.

"We'll make a killing. I can count the millions and we'll all be rich!" decreed the opportunistic head of the firm as he rubbed his hands together in joyful anticipation. (If this were true, why hadn't he and his company done so already instead of many years and lean profits to show for it. There's no such thing as a "free lunch.")

"You can show us how it's done. You've

done it before and this is an easy one," flattered the Board of Directors. They allowed me that denied independence based on my smoothly garbled jargon and seeming well-being. They lost money. I lost much more. I'm truly sorry for the hurt and problems, but I needed guidance and direction, not opportunism and blindness. It's no wonder that I've developed some wisdom and patience.

But, when everything looks the blackest, that's when I found that hope is necessary. Hope and optimism worked wonders for what was to come next.

CHAPTER TEN
"Planning Equals Success"
(George S. May Co. 1980)

The calendar records that many years have passed since this tale began. I'm considerably older now and, I believe, wiser — tempered and honed by the experiences that the life related here provided.. The successes and failures that mold one, the reactions and conclusions that are related here are important footprints to recovery. And they make a place for you and your recovery. From these observations I grew. May you grow, in wisdom and in worth.

The next 10 chapters, essential to the purpose of this book, were first written during and reasonably soon after my stroke of good luck. They comprise the observations, hopefully interesting, not bland and always progressing forward and upward — during the long time of recovery. Reading over and editing some of the unnecessary and sometimes mysterious verbiage I wrote down those many years ago, I realized just how difficult I must have been. (Recently a friend and neighbor reminded me of some of the experiences with our children and me. My friend would just politely listen, nod and grunt when we conversed, never able to understand more than a general essence of what I was trying to say.)

But I also note that my ramblings and jottings always reflected hope, objectivity and forthrightness. They were a diary of sorts and described the mental gymnastics and feelings of that time (generally, the same thoughts and feelings that you may experience) and I believe that they are as alive today as they were then. They express the feelings, attitudes and thinking so essential to continuing life and making a plausible recovery. And, making a better person. They can be a handbook and guide, always with direction. They tell what to expect. They define the thoughts, the expressions of humor, foolishness and always, hope. If the words, the problems, the successes help to provide some answers to questions, assist, guide, clarify the opportunities that life provides, then this effort is well worth it. Time has altered much in life, and progress in medical science has cut the problems and length of time for recovery. But they are the common-sense basics in lay terms.

At times the solutions will seem overly simple. They are. Because when you treat one problem, face one challenge at a time, all your attention and effort for a prolonged period of time is on that problem (that opportunity).. As you progress and make improvement, fix that single problem, all the other concerns like depression or anger or bad stress or pain or whatever, simply go out of your mind and then disappear.

Just follow the directions.

They work!

✓ It starts with an explanation of the medical facts of the situation and an

honest analysis of some physical
ones that apply.

✓ Next, I try to analyze my pain and
pain in general – what it is, kinds,
causes, how to make it bearable
and better.

✓ Depression and despair are easy to
come by, hard to get rid of.

✓ This chapter takes them on with
an examination of the problems, the
symptoms, and possible solutions.

✓ Be forewarned: frustration, anger,
personality alterations and emotions
also "come with the territory."

✓ There can be good and bad stress,
and understanding and handling both
kinds is important.

✓ Learning to face up to a new
existence is critical.

✓ Therapy is necessary to rebuild,
train the body and the mind to
operate acceptably to you and
others.

✓ Examining, learning and
understanding the why and the how
of progress will bring success.

✓ Regaining self-respect and self-
confidence gives you motivation
and direction.

✓ Putting life into perspective, showing
what's necessary and how to
recognize and achieve success.

✓ And, finally, where to go from here?

CHAPTER ELEVEN
"We Try Harder"
(Avis Rent-a-Car, 1962)

What is a stroke?

A stroke occurs when oxygenized blood is suddenly unavailable to the brain. It's like what happens with a heart attack only it's the brain denied the blood and not the heart and that brain suddenly has nothing to work with. The brain cells then systematically die, (necessarily, a simplified analysis.)

There are two kinds of stroke: Ischemic and Hemorrhagic. Those who suffer an Ischemic stroke have either a Cerebral Thrombosis, where a clot is formed near the brain in an artery narrowed by cholesterol or other fatty substance, or a Cerebral Embolism where a clot is formed in another part of the body and travels to the brain and gets lodged there. They say one loses two million brain cells a minute with this kind of stroke and that the second kind is worse. Worse? The second kind is a Hemorrhagic stroke. This type of stroke occurs when a blood vessel bursts open, allowing blood to rush into the brain, itself. Treatment of the two forms is very different and while more deadly, the hemorrhagic stroke is, fortunately, less common.

My stroke was of this latter category,

specifically a Cerebral Hemorrhage, wherein an arterial blood vessel in my brain burst, allowing the blood to rush throughout the brain, systematically destroying it. Once brain cells die, the neural connections are lost and communication and control with the parts of the body cease and the body stops functioning. Right. You're gone, the body's gone, nothing can be saved. Wrong. This is not the end of the story. And, medical discovery now shows that while cells are initially destroyed, they can be repaired. How else to explain me, my physical and mental "rebirth" and abilities — and this book. We'll examine this matter in detail in a later chapter.

What about recovery?

Today, it's believed that partial recovery can be achieved within a year. It took me quite a bit longer. Today we're talking months, not years. Previously accepted medical theory also asserted that if a combination of medicines, machines and therapy can't eliminate the disabilities within a few early months, the disabilities can't be fixed. And, that's wrong, too. They can be fixed. As proof, I'm very much alive, rather a "whole" human being and writing this story for you. The process of regenerating brain cells is called Neurogenesis and regenerating the body is called Neuroplasticity. These are fancy words saying "re-growing brain cells and rewiring and retraining the body to operate" and this story tells why and the how.

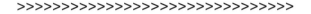

Time has a way of providing perspective. Hours easily slipped into days, weeks into months, months into years. I have faced enough now that I can step back and look honestly at the situation and myself. One must try to do some objective reasoning as to what happens as a result of a calamity and figure out where to go from there. There is an excellent reason for all that guarded medical prognosis. Cold but true — with a cerebral hemorrhage there is an insignificant recovery number. This kind of stroke is deadly. And, if one does make it through, the chances of being a whole person or even a good facsimile are limited, almost non-existent. Any recuperative period is long and frustrating, if at all. But with modern medicine and improved techniques of healing, the time today is a shortened hospital stay and a shortened recuperative period, The prognosis is hopeful. One key to survival and success is speedy action and I can thank Cy and the paramedics and the hospital for that. They say an hour from door to treatment.

But, the other and most important key is you. That's the book is all about.

Initially, I asked myself all the expected questions:

Will I ever be the same person again?

Will I ever be able to live a normal life?

Will I ever have emotions, love, talk right, walk right, work right, function right?

These questions and many more consumed my mind during the long healing process. It was frustrating, all these questions to be answered. I had to mostly answer them myself, for I wasn't able to properly communicate, the mouth not being able to formulate coherent words to others, let alone accept the usual "everything will be fine," or "things don't look too good, do they?"

The head hurt but thankfully the pain was deadened by the nerve damage. There was despair in all the questions — like what's in store, what's going to happen to me? Was I mixed up, messed up?

OK, I've got lots of time — they can be clinical. So can I.

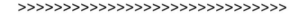

Let's divide the problems into some sort of order.

Speech

Mine was an acute case of not speaking clearly and not being able to communicate the thoughts that were formed in my head. I think it was about six months before I experienced real improvement. (More about improvement – time, stages, plateaus is treated a bit later in the book.) I did rather poorly in those early stages of my new world, then better. Technically, I think it was a loss of coordination and thus communication between what was the thought and how the brain interpreted and relayed to what came out of my mouth. Practically, this was a probably a matter of the tongue and the lips not being able to form the speech that normal brain impulses would transmit. Like a baby. (Remember seeing those movies where the baby's thoughts are verbalized in the audio?) I sounded as if I had a mouthful of mush or as if I had drunk too much alcohol or was on drugs. The nurses used to gather in a frustrated and argumentative group, unaware of my antennae being able to overhear and comprehend their comments: "Can't understand a word he says," or "How do we know what to do, how does the doctor prescribe treatment if we can't get a feedback on what it does, whether it hurts, whether it works?," Or frustrated, "He just lies there, can't talk, can't walk," Or, "The food's OK, but he can't seem to get it down..." All those positive little comments that I didn't need to hear. I rapidly developed a hard veneer through it all and used it all as a challenge to correct the problems.

Motor Control (and body parts)

Walking was a problem. "Perambulation" may have been a better word because "motion of sorts" best described my initial efforts. I "walked" with a list toward the affected right side (when I walked at all). Crawling, staggering may have been better descriptions. This lasted about a year. Motor control — there was none. Simply, there was little or no brain communication to the body's motor function. Needed lots of that "rewiring." My left hand had almost no control.

I still can't play the piano, and it was 10 years before I could hold anything liquid in my left hand. Other more easily hidden (and now mostly controlled problems) were lack of balance, caused by that impaired motor function, and the paralyzed nerves and stomach entry that affected eating and swallowing functions.

Rewiring this body of mine is going to take a long time and be pretty taxing and frustrating. All I can do is keep trying, pushing, new things, find out what works and what doesn't.

Regaining motor skills is so much shorter, easier and better today with the help of knowledge and experience (and something called physical therapy). There were other, smaller, but bothersome concerns .and we'll look at them later.

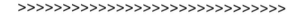

Symptoms may vary, day-to-day. There were, there are going to be, serious physical and mental limitations. The mind might not work well one day, the body the next. One day may be better than before or the next. But I'm getting ahead of things. Once I was first awake, physically if not mentally, I felt that all must be OK and acted the part. I didn't, wouldn't comprehend, understand that I was still a very sick individual. This (escapism) was the basis for all the rest of the mental problems I encountered. But you have to go there to make it right. All the things these chapters treat are the result of my "leaving the door open" for all of the mental "ambushes"

that awaited me. Trial and error. It goes on for quite a while, taxing the family and concerned others as well as me. I had to remember that the family and those closest bear a tremendous amount of pressure. I'm taken care of, but who takes care of them while the major problems are handled, serious effects neutralized?

I progressed rapidly at first, overcoming many obstacles, the obstacles that we'll look at later in detail. Then progress became slower, less defined. It's a wonder that I still had a wife, friends. With all I had a simple and child-like response and, as a result, a similar relationship. It took time to realize this fact, recognize the slowness of progress and its subtleties. My thoughts and actions were complex and clumsy and it's probably just as well that I couldn't really discern all of that going on because I'd be mortified and hiding from the facts.

Proper association with others then is of vital importance and assistance. It was primarily through this assistance and association with life that I progressed beyond immediate personal concerns and began to develop outwardly. This is the essential first step in recovery. And, recovery is a demanding, taxing experience for everyone and provides seemingly insurmountable problems. Recovery is then limited by the quantity and quality of the cure (the care received) — namely, the people, their input, their actions and reactions. All of this probably sounds a bit cold and clinical but the facts are necessary to get to and understand the truth. I tried to look at myself, at it all, in a factual and objective way. Sure feelings have a place.

I'm not an overtly emotional type but more than once or twice I choked-up, shed a few tears, realized that what is, is not forever and if I didn't pull myself up by the bootstraps, then whatever people did for me wasn't going to make a hill 'o beans and I'd wallow in self-pity and never make it back. The point here is simple: I'm alive because I've learned to be a better person in spite of and because of my infirmities. An old saying, but adversity does have a way of bringing out the best. I had to fight for the morals of life and it began to dawn on me just how important they are. Without honesty I couldn't face and solve all my problems, my dilemmas. Integrity forced me to look realistically at matters both good and bad and try a little harder.

And, I was damned afraid !

CHAPTER TWELVE
"Snap, Crackle, Pop"
(Kellogg Cereals, 1939)

I hurt physically and mentally because pain is both. It's more: whether the result of operation or cataclysmic trauma, your body is going to rebel. And that's pain.

What does it mean? The dictionary describes pain as "a disturbing sensation resulting from injurious external interference." Rather obtuse and cold for what I was feeling. Better: "unpleasant, unbearable, annoying, suffering, aching, clinging, grasping, untenable — and damn, It hurts!" In medical language, pain is a soreness or tenderness over some particular part of the body. Pain may be localized where the problem occurred, or sympathetic, where pain appears in other parts of the body. than where the injury or invasion occurred. And when the body is invaded by whatever means and its well-tuned function is disrupted, there's going to be a reaction. Called pain. Someone once said that pain can control our actions, our lives.

Practically, there are three different kinds of pain: sharp pain — like sticking in a knife, maybe making it worse by turning it, or dull pain, where it's a constant, annoying ache and mental pain, where one hurts wherever because one is supposed to hurt wherever. Hold on, I thought, maybe there's some truth hiding here. Athletes ignore pain, endure it, play through it. So the brain can be an ally, helping. So maybe I can train the brain? So maybe I could play it this way and turn pain into a positive to make me work harder and better? And eventually the brain could ignore and adapt? And the pain would be better. (Just hoped there was enough "brain" there to do it, all we can do is try...)

I think I experienced them all. On a scale of 1-10, there were times when it was a 10. But mostly it was an unpleasant, unbearable, annoying, suffering, dull, constant ache of a 4 or 5. But I was lucky, the pain was bearable because I fortunately couldn't feel a lot of it. The electrical system was semi-inoperative, deadened so that the pain seemed less severe, just the usual short-term shocks, long-term aches. Sometimes the pain kept up, hour after hour, day after day. I wondered how I could tolerate it. I wondered, and my mind wandered: *this is what Hell must be like?*

I finally concluded that pain should be compared with trying to sleep at night and having to listen to a dripping faucet. It drips the same. Constantly. But the noise seems to get louder and louder until you can't stand it and you can't sleep, (counting sheep doesn't help, no matter how many sheep.) The body cries out for sleep, only the mind repeats — "drip, drip, drip." All leads to a ruined body and a ruined mind. I became irritable, irrational, tired and nasty.

And, I could see the results — depression, affecting physical being and bodily function. It had started. Not for me. That wasn't what I was, not what I wanted to be. Depression, that's the problem and solution in the next chapter.

Pain can also be worse with an injury to the brain, because that's the center of things. Such traumas are a momento of war or accident. There are hundreds of young men and women returning home after serving their country, wounded in battle, wounded in life, mind and spirit. And everyday life can turn into a battle, too.

That's what this book is about, and why, neurological brain damage. Whether it's stroke, injury, Alzheimers, Parkinsons, MS, palsy, autism, arthritis, war injury, life's injury — whatever, the list goes on. It's called hard work and hope. But we're getting ahead of ourselves.—we're just getting started.

So, before any concern, before any depression, despair, eventual stress interfering with any meaningful recovery, I knew that I had to level with the doctors, the caregivers, about the "what" and the "where" of the pain, even if it seemed everywhere at once. They might be able to figure it out. They did. It was the wiring, my nerves misfiring. It was like a series of electric shocks and shorts and it better be fixed before there was a fire. Sure, there are drugs and pills to fix the problem — temporarily. But I felt that I needed to go beyond the muscles and the bones and fix the "invisible" — the nerves and the mind. That's why I was reviewing and trying to analyze this mess, called me. I concentrated my thoughts on the positives, that the end result of a "well me" would be worth all the suffering and seemingly eternal misery, the pangs, the aches, the torment.

And I thought: *In life there had been hurt to get where I was going, but the end result was a better me. So, do it here. It's worth more if one has to fight for it, struggle for it because achieving the goal then means something that is not only satisfying, but lasting.*

I found that by knowing and doing these things, the pain became easier to handle and eventually disappeared entirely.

One down, many to go. Was I up to the task of handling all the other problems? The mental challenges had to come first as they'd make it easier to figure out the physical mess I was in.

One at a time.

Next?

CHAPTER THIRTEEN
"Wonder Where The Yellow Went?"
(Pepsodent Toothpaste, 1953)

Despair was the first real emotion that I recognized. It pervaded my slowly awakening mind. It was a feeling of utter hopelessness and discouragement. What could I do? Anything? There are other appropriately descriptive words like emptiness, uselessness, despondency. And depression — and I was depressed! This sounds terrible but it appropriately described my state of mind, state of being. I hadn't gotten to desperation yet. That would come later.

I tried to look at my situation and make some sense out of it, and of myself, and in this case, thought a bit of rationalizing might just work well. And, I tried.

A word I used earlier to describe my feelings was discouragement, and that's the result of disappointment or rejection or failure. Well, I thought, that didn't apply because I hadn't yet had time for any failures. Rejection — the hospital took good care of that, always doing things to me, for me, no rejection or disappointment, just their way. Hopelessness? Oh, yes, early on. But since I hadn't had any discouragements yet in my recuperation efforts (we're not talking about my whole life becoming a shambles — we're just looking at the ways of turning it around, making it, me, better) then I couldn't be facing the hopelessness that results. Anyway, hopelessness is negative and I didn't need any negative feelings. And that would lead to apathy and a lack of hope, and despair would result from this abandoning of hope and is going to bring with it sadness and distress. No way. I had to keep on hoping. Something to "hang my hat on, hold on to." So, I wasn't desperate because desperation is no more than energized despair, resulting in vigorous and reckless actions and consequences. So, hope is all I had, and I had to hold on. Boy, I really was analyzing and rationalizing.

OK.

Back up — I'm depressed.

What's it mean? It means saddened, dejected, weakened.

Who's sad? The hospital, my family are doing their best for me so why shouldn't I? Dejected? That's the clearest route to self-pity and I saw no need because that would mean giving up hope and the chance at making some progress out of this dismal, almost retarded state. Weakened? That's physical and I also instinctively felt that I could get better. I'm living and more or less functioning and that's an improvement over the alternative.

Depression has no place, and suddenly I found that I had talked myself around it.

So, my earlier moments were accompanied by feelings of uselessness and frustration, and I was in a despondent and forlorn state of mind. I was distressed goods. Being the optimist has its advantages (if I only could have foreseen some of the future problems, I might have reconsidered). Doesn't it all reflect that earlier episode about waking up, coming to "life," uncertain of what and who I was? It's easy to settle into a despondent state of mind, accept a chronic dejection. And I experienced all of this at one time or another during the course of my recovery.

But, forewarned is forearmed. It needn't be all bad. I used it as a motivation to strive for better, for more of what I wanted to come back to, come back to be. But I had to constantly remind myself that self-analysis and conscious preparation is fine, but I had to also keep telling myself, over and over, what was needed, what I had to do, wanted to do, think and be.

Always remember that nothing in this life is free. It all comes with a price tag. You've got to be willing to "pay the piper," as they say. When it got too bad, I just thought of it all as a military battle, to gain ground, a little piece here and there, akin to getting those little pieces of my life back again. And these little victories were going to result in ultimately winning the war. I was up to it because the end result was worth it.

I had to constantly remind myself of what and where and how it was and how I wanted it to be and how I knew it could be.

In summary: Despair leads to all kinds of problems on the long road to nowhere. Depression leads to weakness, and I knew better than to go down that path. Despondency leaves one unable to function properly. Discouragement leads to not trying. Desperation makes for irrational and mostly unsatisfying activity. I needed direction, but direction guided by those with my best interests at heart. It was fortunate for me that I heeded the wisdom and experience of those around me, tempered by what I, in my gut, instinctively knew was best. The key was to face whatever problems head-on with the best knowledge and best thinking that I could muster at the time. Then approach them honestly, openly, realistically. It worked. The problems resolved themselves.

These wanderings and meanderings with a little psychology and practicality thrown in are just that. But this was really the first time that I could honestly say I was thinking and analyzing.

CHAPTER FOURTEEN
"Sometimes You Feel
Like A Nut"
(Peter Paul Candy Bars, 1953)

Frustration comes easily with a stroke. It comes easily with any illness or injury, surgery or severe complication to routine. Webster's tells it in big words: Frustration means something being done for naught, its purpose, repeatedly defeated. Practically, it meant to me that to avoid frustration in whatever, I had to take one small step at a time, and then stop and savor the result. Progress was worth the effort and whatever time it took. Handle each problem as I recognized it. Experience and a voice inside wisely told me that a lack of progress was going to be a problem with which I was not yet ready to cope and I'd better realize the restrictions "up front" and that even, slow and steady steps, taken one at a time, would result in accomplishment and eventually bring its own reward.

Another real danger to any recovery was becoming self-centered. Through trail and error I had found that any activity centered around gratifying only me and forget anyone else, wouldn't really work for me. So, in the beginning I experienced selfishness and exaggerated stubbornness with an attitude of righteousness thrown in. I tried to disguise it all by acting the opposite, attempting what was supposed to be improbable, often even impossible. This was in order to draw praise and exhort sympathy. All it did was complicate things, including my life. This would eventually lead to a personality change and I don't think I wanted that. And that's not what all of this was about. If I were to make a recovery it had better be a good recovery and a better me. Otherwise what was the sense in all of this, why the struggle, why the suffering, why the pain, why the effort unless the result was a better person? So much for self, and selfishness.

And then there was that third personality problem, one that beat inside of me to get out. Many times it did. Not so bad, it's called "letting off steam," and it was probably caused by that old nemesis, frustration. The books call it "anger" and I call it stupid. But looking back objectively, it was only natural to experience resentment, indignation, anger at this unwanted tragedy. Sure, I was mad at the world. At times I would seethe inside at the unfairness. And I was often very emotional, as this anger boiled over. Result? It got me nowhere. And it was rather embarrassing.

CHAPTER FIFTEEN
"You Deserve A Break Today"
(McDonalds Restaurants, 1971)

The media talks about the mental and physical concern we call stress. Back when all this started, stress didn't exist as a term for anything except something in mechanical engineering. I had read a little, heard some about mental anguish and the physical problems that could result, but I was woefully unprepared for the totality of my own feelings and actions. The main problem seemed to be emotional and was mostly determined by my simple interpretation of the problems and questions facing me. This distress was not necessarily a natural thing, rather an influence that made me do things compulsively.

Stress came easily with this territory - it was so easy to get "up-tight" or "stressed-out," to use today's vernacular. My situation cried out for stress because it stimulated me. Which leads to a question and an early-on concern: There's a whole new concept that there's good stress, too.

Stress can also be a natural thing, forcing change and adaptation and stress keeps you on your toes, to live a healthy, functional life.

How could I tell the difference, and did it

make a difference?

At first I was in denial about any kind of stress. Oh, not me, the easy-going one. While much depended on my previous personality and actions, there was change. My situation went beyond the "good stress." As shown earlier, I was irritable, short and abrupt with others and with myself. I tried to do everything at once, certainly more than that for which I was mentally and physically capable of handling. Especially at the time   Relationships were important but they were influenced by my moods and behavior. People would pick-up on my actions and be influenced by my rants and ravings and all it accomplished was to make everyone edgy, short and upset. But stress, good or bad, is determined by the interpretation of a situation. Stress management has to start with the problem — me. To correct my problems I decided that I had to start at the beginning. (time was a commodity in long supply). So I would draw a picture, a diagram, in my mind, displaying the concerns and their necessary solutions and try to make steady and tangible progress in my actions and my decisions. Frustration, despair, pain could be faced and conquered, one at a time. No mean feat. I told myself that I needed to make steady visible progress. Slow, but avoid failure. That would take care of the bad stress. It did. And it developed a lot of the patience necessary to avoid the pitfalls of trying to do too much, too soon. That would do nothing but bring back all the bad stress I had shed. The good stress would remain to push me towards a proper recovery. So, bad stress wasn't scary anymore, and it became just another obstacle conquered along the way to living a real life again.

Now, I knew I was on the right track.

CHAPTER SIXTEEN
"This Is Your Brain.
This Is Your Brain On Drugs."
(Partnership for a Drug-Free America, 1987)

It's important to look at the major problems that resulted from all these emotional difficulties, and, to question the mistakes.   A serious trauma makes the adrenaline flow and the ego grow. I put on a performance that overtly hid the pain, disguised the facts, and covered-up the difficulties and the problems. These actions seemed timely and appropriate to me, proper, lucid, correct.

Far from it — I needed help. My help, and help from the people around me, the professionals and those who just cared. But I had to learn — the hard way.

The first problem varies in degree from person to person.   It's one of personality change. What is personality? It's that which constitutes what and who we are. Let's go back a bit in time. Psychologists tell us that, with the exception of trauma, an individual's personality traits are established by the time they are 6 and remain consistent throughout their life. I had been traumatized and my "personality" reflected it. I tried to make some sense out of this strange new "me." Was it an ego thing, a result of being subjected to new obstacles, new challenges, new stimuli? Was it a subconscious reliance on past experience and ability, grasping at the familiar, no threat, no menace? Outside circumstances and my environment, must have affected the change. My major problem was in establishing an identity — necessary. But in this lay a trap and a challenge: be who I was, be my age, with the stature of experience and knowledge. I wasn't ready. So, I showed bad judgment and made mistakes. But with supervision and input from others I think I managed, pretty well. Psychoanalysis came with this new territory and I was smart enough to know that the professionals knew more than I. It made it easier to absorb and learn.

The next problem was physical. Forget about matters of walking, speaking, eating, we already know about them. My errors were of trying too hard, too soon. I was beginning to feel better and act better, but I really wasn't. Heretofore hidden attributes and negatives were exposed. I couldn't hide. My physical strength was enhanced, my mental capabilities, sapped. I will always remember some of my behavior, humorous now but at the time embarrassing and potentially damaging, While ostensibly repairing a water outlet, I became angry and proceeded to rip the faucet and accompanying pipes from the wall. Strength seemed to increase in inverse proportion to my ability. But, "carefully" was not then a word in my vocabulary. Watch out. I tackled simple carpentry around the house. It used to be so easy. Oh, yes, everything was done — at an angle. At least it worked. Electric endeavors usually ended in shock therapy as my left hand just wouldn't function. Plumbing exercise just wasn't even on the horizon. There were other outward examples of misdirected prowess, perhaps in pain, perhaps in reaction, perhaps in frustration. The point of the matter is that it was a subconscious thing, appropriate to the new (and fortunately temporary) personality guiding the body and whatever meager thinking that would come. Although I thought I was brilliant, in reality I was a clown without makeup, as appropriate one who delighted in getting a laugh.

Another problem was the loss of the ability to properly reason. Reason is the basis for intelligent action. And, mine was somewhat warped. I took this simple, everyday process for granted; for it was natural. Any illness, any surgery, however, is going to affect the body and it's going to affect the mind, cause changes in the normal pattern of life.

I lost this ability to reason. Forever, I thought, but I gradually learned that it was only temporarily retarded. I learned that reasoning may seem sound to the "reasoner" but not necessarily rational to the observer. I learned that mistakes may be small or large or may not seem like mistakes at all   But they may later result in serious problems and have disastrous consequences, if they are not recognized by someone trusted and shown in their true vein. But, sometimes loved ones wanted to pacify me, "baby" me. Forgive a little preaching from one who's been there. There's a fine line between maximum personal effort and too much. Only those who care the most, in this case, my spouse knew what that line was. She'd been through it with me before, knew the boundaries of reasonable achievement, understood and could recognize my limits. And she pushed (how many times did I feel like pushing back, I'd be so damned angry, really hiding disgust with myself.) Bless you, Nancy, for you wouldn't let me give up, pushing me to push harder, achieve, more and better.

Those who matter the most, care the most and must be "tough," seemingly cold and callous. It made me work harder and try harder and see success, for once I saw it, lived it — I wanted more. It's difficult, but so necessary. In later years, teaching classes to victims of strokes and tragic illnesses, I saw the truth and satisfaction on the much bigger stage of life. In the vernacular, it's called "tough love". Facing up to my problems was, is important. But, I also learned caution and I found through trial and error that presenting a situation or challenge, a problem of real consequence, was not yet desirable. I thought that by now I'd be ready. I felt ready. I wasn't. I still needed that guidance and "tough love." It's probably the hardest single area that I and those who cared for me had to cope.

One incident will always remind me of this. Left to my own resources one day after the hospitals when my spouse finally felt comfortable getting some breathing room away from the "patient": "Don't go where you haven't been before, where you can't physically handle problems, especially out back and don't go near the hill because you have no balance and it's dangerous for you..."

So what did I do?   Climbed up that hill, to get something or just prove a point, I don't remember. (Now you know one of the reasons why I survived: strong-willed, stubborn, willing to accept the consequences of trial and error, good physical condition) What happened? I fell. Hard. To the asphalt drive. Luckily, I wasn't dead, just badly bruised. The body would heal, the bruised ego, too. If I had only listened, thought it through. A lesson.

There were other problems that had to be turned into opportunities to get better. Little by little, I improved, learned to adapt, to do thoughtful and practical things. My spirit and the physical and unique thing called my body was still there, and it was beginning to "come around" and function. I had to constantly remind myself that for whatever their reasons, motivations and interests, the doctors, nurses, wife and children, family, friends, people whose lives let me in — all had something to give and teach and It was up to me to put it into my personal computer For the brain was inching forward in some sort of "recovery" mode and I knew that I could make it all work for a new and improved version of me.

My damage was centered in the brain. It was a sudden, powerful, debilitating debacle that affected the brain and my nervous and circulatory systems. Repair to this kind of damage is possible only if it is accomplished with great patience and care — on everyone's part. I had to live a very regulated existence in a very small, minutely controlled world. I yearned for the things I did before and could no longer do. I was an athlete and now sports and athletic endeavors were forbidden. I loved music and I could no longer sing or play the piano, only listen. I had a quick and incisive mind and I could now only stammer poorly-formed and awkward thoughts and those very slowly. I had been an adult, a rather competent, capable, caring person with responsibilities and a well-earned place in society.

Then, in an instant, I was transformed into a child and at first, really an infant, a dependant, diaper-wearing, mewling infant, crawling around. A friend recently pointed out just how important that child-like state was to recovery. The infant, the child is self-centered, focused on feelings of being warm, comfortable, safe and secure, being fed, kept clean. They rest all the time because the body only grows when they are asleep. They manipulate their environment to their needs, repeating things over and over until they master a new skill. They control others in simple ways like crying, pleasing smiles and "baby talk." And, they have all the time in the world. As did I. Take time. Being a "baby" is not a problem, it is the necessary healing pattern with which one must begin.

Sure, I lamented what was lost, but I was beginning to appreciate and look for that something that was better than what was.

And, it was coming.

CHAPTER SEVENTEEN
"Be All That You Can Be"
(U.S. Army/N.W. Ayer, 1981)

One of the first activities they allow you in hospitals these days is physical therapy. The salutary effects of physical endeavor weren't even considered when I was entombed in a hospital bed. It was rest and treatment. Then, therapy was only considered something involved in the treatment of whatever condition.. It was concerned with the discovery, application and action of medicines and remedies for illness, simply, the art of healing. Since then, we have learned the salutary affects of a healthy body, ergo physical endeavor, therapy and what it is today. The old sports axiom of "no pain, no gain" is the result and is paramount to recovery. I walked, I exercised under supervision. With help, I fine-tuned my body until it began to work reasonably well.

I constantly reminded myself of how the physical being is built and organized. Relating to my communications past, I put it in practical terms and codompared my body to a radio or television station. I compared my body to prthat of the production of programs where the brain became the Master Control. We've seen this scene depicted in the movies and on the television. Or perhaps you're a sports fan and can relate all this to a professional football game. Other sports follow the same general pattern. but with football the closeups and action sequences are more graphic (stay tuned, we're going somewhere).

Each camera is focused on a piece of the whole and that picture is transmitted to a panel of pictures on screens and this Master Control provides for a selection from the whole of whatever picture the Director, he or she, feels is required at the time. To relate further, from this Master Control (the brain) impulses travel through an organized maze of wires and electronic impulses hooked up to the working parts of the production (the body). There are subsidiary or small control rooms for each production studio, just as there area for centers of strategic locations for parts of the body to control individual and delegated functions. Damage a working part of the studio or production (cameras, relays, screens, etc.) and it has to be fixed. Be it bone, muscle or "wiring," the body's the same. Doctors, nurses, hospitals all worked to fix what was mechanically wrong, mostly trying to make better what was lost or damaged, using medicines to help the process. But back to the television studio — I was the Director and I had to make the decision on what camera, what picture. (Today, it's probably easier with the Internet and wireless features, but I'm certain the concept is the same and, besides, medicine, technology, has advanced so much.

But it's the psychological and emotional that I am relating on these pages and how it all works together.

I strained, I sweated, and I sometimes cried

out from the exertion and the pain but I forced myself with the control, and the experience of trial and error. Behind all this effort is the motivation to succeed or I wouldn't be here writing this story.

A caution: I found that my mental attitude toward the therapy had everything to do with its success. I focused on the end result, endured the regularity, the drudgery, sometimes the boredom, the exertion, the tears. It was a long, hard way, and a job, if you will — to reach a goal. How much, how long depends on the severity of the matter. But the end result was my necessary goal. It's easy, now, to look back and think of the sacrifice. It was a tedious route to the glorious end of a competent person ready to meet and conquer the challenges of life. And, I must constantly remind myself of the problems, the sacrifices that I made, others made and the help that was given.

Which all leads to an appropriate and happy tale of an accomplished young lady – and a runner.

She was in her early 20s. She was a competitive gymnast in her high school years. She graduated to distance running in college. Improved it in grad school. She was determined and a bit stubborn, wouldn't give up, pressed and constantly upped her endurance, even when it must have hurt. She won many an event but her finest effort came under duress, when, in spite of physical problems, she finished third in a field of thousands.

It was my good fortune to run with this young lady. It was some time after those many hospitals. I was better, physically, mostly. But my endurance wasn't up to the challenge yet and lack of balance complicated the effort. She left me huffing and puffing and with the constant memory of being so very out of shape and not being able to push, go that "extra mile." So much for continuing therapy, I thought, then forgetting that it was a mental necessity as well. Yet, out of every experience comes something good. It taught me that physical exertion, continued exercise was still necessary to long-term recovery, to function, to live a life as a parent, a husband, a responsible and effective person. .

Life presented the why. Mental therapy led me to know the physical.

Shelley, my youngest daughter, had shown me the way.

CHAPTER EIGHTEEN
"Catch Our Smile"
(PSA Airlines 1968)

Learning from my children was not new to me. And I recall a particular breakfast table discussion many years ago. As usual it was a meaningful discussion and somehow got around to my work, advertising and how it could help everyone, including my family.

"OK, here's the situation," I challenged. The family always seemed to put its best mind to work at mealtime. After all, nourishment helps the whole body work together (that's this whole story) and meal times are really family togetherness times. We always did things as a family because we had learned in our East Coast sojourn that while money builds a house, love and family build a home — and a life.

"There's this client that's been with my new advertising firm for a while. It's a very popular airline, PSA. Now, we're going to try television ads for getting their message out to more people for less money. You remember Maslov, "message before medium" — well, we have the message and we know the medium, but the problem is: how do we do the creative part? .

"What are they doing now, Daddy?" Shelley, the youngest daughter, asked. "And, does it work?"

I replied, "It's print, newspaper and magazine. They have a message and a method that works very well. They show pictures of the airplane, talk about comfort and service, good-looking stewardesses in good-looking outfits to care for the passengers, emphasizing the speed of travel, low fares, etc. And they put a smiling face on the airplane to show the plane's satisfaction with it all and that's the tone of the copy. That, of course, translates into passenger satisfaction to the potential customer reading the ad.

"Oh, Dad," interjected the oldest girl, Lisa, "It's so obvious, and simple. You just put the smile on the pictures of the airplane in the television commercials and put that same smile on the real planes. They've got to like it because it just makes sense. It does what you've been saying, and it's so easy. You taught us well. You can convince them. I know you can."

I did. The key was having the airplane smile. And we put a real smile on the airline because that simple idea helped them fly successfully and profitably for many years.

And, what I was learning through my ordeal was that a smile works on a person's face just as well as it does on the face of an airplane.

CHAPTER NINETEEN
"Keeps Going and Going and Going"
(Energizer Batteries, 1986)

Recovery takes a good while. Recovery comes in a series of stages. I struggled to reach an objective, had to remain happy with that achievement for a good while, during which time nothing seemed to move or change much at all. Liken it to climbing, onward, upward, then a resting place, a level place, a plateau where the body regroups, recuperates, acquires new strength, preparing itself before "climbing" to the next level, the next level of wellness.

Progress came quickly in the beginning, then slowly. In the early stages of recovery the body often made dramatic leaps of improvement, happening forcefully, readily, quickly. Then everything seemed to slow down. Sometimes, very slowly, and frustrating is too kind a word, boring too harsh. But all the time, and no back sliding, the body was regrouping, making things better. And as long as there was recognizable progress, this slow pace was acceptable. I struggled to achieve an objective. Not all at once but one step, one thing at a time, and I forced myself to remain happy with that accomplishment. I took heart from all this when I realized that whatever progress, however small or slow, it was always steady and upward. I saw that the end result would be good and I couldn't dwell on the downside. I found that by trial and error and the passage of time, another step forward was taken, painstakingly prepared by nature, and I could see a new and higher place was in the offing. It was slow, but I could feel and see progress.

And the whole thing became a play, a drama in which there were five acts of personal growth to be realized, to be acted out in each Stage of Progress. It's like growing up — again.

- ✓ The <u>FIRST STAGE</u> was the most difficult for a grown adult because it's a physical and mental reversion in actions and thought to the stage of an infant (we've explored this in some detail in an earlier chapter.)

- ✓ Next came the <u>SECOND STAGE</u>, that of a child, a juvenile and most often selfish state of being. This one was also hard to stomach, and my way of handling it (and life) was awkward by any standard.

- ✓ The <u>THIRD STAGE</u> was a graduation to early youth with all of its problems. I'd gone through adolescence once, but now I had the maturity of years and the experience of life to guide and that of others to lead. (Read "Zits" on the comics page of your local newspaper and you'll understand.) Easier for me but often hard for those around me.

✓ Soon, the <u>FOURTH STAGE</u> of young adulthood and I've tried to convey the highlights, the progress and the rush of success that resulted.

✓ Wait, cried the voice of conscience — most decisions still had to be made for me or were influenced by others. Too soon, and attempts at personal and professional business were bumbling and ineffective. Responsibilities of life were still something of a nuisance. Most rational feelings and affection were something beyond me. I still tried to function as I thought others desired. It doesn't work. But the strong desire to take a rightful place often obscures what is right or needed. Take care, don't rush it, as it will come.

✓ And, the rightful conclusion to this play, wherein you make your own happy ending is the fifth and final act. I did. It's the <u>FIFTH STAGE</u> of a mature adult with wisdom and vision that this experience teaches. Often beyond my years, it's an awesome challenge and equal responsibility.

And, there are necessary steps to make all this work.

CHAPTER TWENTY
"From Experience Comes Faith"
(E. R. Squibb & Sons, 1961)

Go back to the beginning. You're lying there, staring vacantly at that sterile ceiling, maybe focusing on that light that mostly works. Maybe a hospital, maybe a home, it makes no difference.

You're down, you wonder why, and you hurt. You think: *Maybe if I had a gun, I'd end it all."*

Take heart, you don't need to go down that road.

Everyone's different, and everyone has different problems, different needs and different wants.

I thought I was the only one in the world in my situation, with my difficulties, and my limited experience said that it was only going to get worse mentally.

Wrong.

A stroke involves the mental and the physical, actions and attitudes and the extent of the problems depend on what kind of stroke and how one handles the seriousness of the matter and understands the possibilities of recovery. In earlier chapters I tried to look at and analyze what happened to me, look at the kinds of strokes and how they affected the body and mind. I had to continually remind and examine

mine, and me, in order to measure advance and progress. But what follows can apply to other kinds of brain damage, injury or brain disorders like Parkinsons, Alzheimers.

With my stroke, physical as well as mental ability was destroyed, resulting in first wholesale then partial paralysis. There was a tremendous need for rest and recuperation from any exertion, and it far exceeded the norm. Speech suffered, slurred from the trauma and exertion and speaking also resulted in mental tiredness. My hand shook; it and the body wouldn't perform or cooperate in coordination matters. A lack of proper function in my legs, arms, head and body carriage were things that frustrated. I felt beyond discouragement. I had to fight against that vicious whirlpool of depression that most often resulted – remember that earlier chapter, about the way to handle and avoid?

So, I began to think, in broader terms :

Isn't physical limitation more important to the afflicted than the observer?

Over and over, I had to repeat:

It's my ego that's bruised. It's going to get better, be better, if I just keep trying, again and again.

And, I'm not alone, the symptoms may be different, some better, some worse, but all of this applies to any devastating, physical difficulty.

And I said to myself:

Self, just be thankful that you can put your feet under you and feel the floor each morning as you climb out of bed. Be thankful for another day, another chance. And when those legs don't work, remember the man who has no legs...

By trial and error I learned that physical activities always appear easier until you try to do them. Compare it to climbing a ladder. You look at what seems simple, normal, and start out with great confidence and normal speed. No way. With the first step your foot quivers, your hand is unsure. So you proceed carefully, slowly, clinging to every support. As you go up that ladder, you become more sure of yourself. Confidence builds. The support is still there but you begin to rely on it less — and less. It all gets more comfortable and secure and then easier and easier. That's how it is with life and that's how recovery works. I had to be adventurous, I had to be investigative; I had to question; I had to have patience; I had to be persistent. I had to try over and over and over until I got it right or, at least, acceptable. What else? This was an obligation because I was given a second chance to redo me from a narrow and materialistic life — the right way.

I will always remember this admonition by a professor in college: "One man's tears are another's lesson." Yes, I'd had those tears, and with them learned how to handle most situations.

So, here's the "dead" man's EIGHT STEPS TO RECOVERY AND RENOVATION:

✓ <u>STEP ONE:</u> Reduce pampering and self-pity and take positive actions. In other words, "stand-up and be counted" and take responsibility, for good or ill — block-out any insecurity and know that it's going to be good.

✓ <u>STEP TWO:</u>   Develop positive mental attitudes and actions that convey present day philosophy and activity. "Get with it." (This was hard because I don't understand a lot in this new and different world and living in the past was security.) Music, reading, television, computers, I-phones, whatever it takes. Relating with children and with young people, trying to understand.   It makes life a lot easier.

✓ <u>STEP THREE:</u> Remember that mental gymnastics will properly follow physical well-being.   Understand the body and don't baby it.   I had to concentrate on making this scenario possible, so I set up a calisthenics (or whatever other physical therapy necessary) routine. According to the U.S. Dept. of Health statistics, exercise lowers the risk of stroke by 27 per cent. If it worked that well to prevent stroke, then I felt it could work to help with rewiring and recovery. Worth a try. And, it worked. I followed the routine faithfully. Even when I was tired. I adjusted. Even when it was inconvenient. I instigated a more healthy diet, eating regular and balanced meals. Importantly, I was sensible about it.   I also learned a lot about dietary problems and that much has to do with genes and metabolism.

✓ <u>STEP FOUR:</u> Regain normality in life

as quickly as possible. I reduced the amount of rest and made those "awake" hours count for more. I forced myself to retire at a regular hour and rise at a regular hour each morning just as I did in my earlier working years.

✓ STEP FIVE: Speak, read out loud. I spoke with groups, spoke in public. I took hold and tried to live a normal existence, with the confusion, the complications, the responsibilities of life. And a life that is right for today. I, not the experts, had to satisfy the ultimate critic — me. I had to take a great deal of care. I still have to take a great deal of care. It's worth it.

✓ STEP SIX: Learn new things, particularly in the areas of business, politics and economics. I discovered that by stimulating my mind, educating myself in these areas, I found ways to better the old. Once learned, I found that I could practice and improve on this new knowledge by teaching it to others. Me, a "sick" man, teaching myself, then teaching these new and better ways to others. It helped me to become whole again.

✓ STEP SEVEN: Listen to and follow medical advice I'm not going to climb mountains, scuba dive or win athletic events. There are physical restrictions, more serious at first, fewer as the years went by, as I began to adapt to a new way of living. I knew when I was ready for whatever because I experimented with simple physical activities. It wasn't really that hard and not really so bad. At first, it seemed a tragedy. (A small price to pay.) Then things got easier. I could do things I supposedly couldn't do. It's rather like school, like arithmetic, putting two and two together to equal four not three. I found that complete compliance was necessary in the beginning, (fudging came later as I made progress). I had to forget any participation in many activities because they inherently presented a physical risk to my body, to my psyche and to others. No more could I do things that required mental and physical coordination, like tennis or like surveying the world from atop a high peak before plummeting downward on those two wooden boards (skis, in those days). Besides, any attempt at these things was often ludicrous. But there are compensatory endeavors like fishing, camping, swimming (a great activity to enhance your physical well-being and improve your coordination) and golf. The latter is a great mental and physical activity — and it's better to walk on top of the grass than underneath it.

✓ STEP EIGHT: This is the simplest. It's reading and learning about medical advances, life today, triumphs of man against adversity. People and politics. Learning about activities that interest and that I might be able to do, the avocations and hobbies that might allow me to be better, do better and achieve better.

CHAPTER TWENTY-ONE
"Think"
(IBM, 1914)

"Think Different"
(Apple Computer/Chiat-Day, 1998)

As if there weren't already enough to think about, practice, do, stages to expect, steps to take (but then, there's a lot of time to think and practice) — here are three more, important tips for obtaining "wellness."

✓ LISTEN
I learned what it was like. To really listen and digest what others said and did. It's really easy. And, it's educating. I observed actions, hard at first, but so important to my learning about others, about me. I listened to my physicians who could provide the best that medical science offered. Sure, I had to open up my life for the professional to see and advise but it was up to me to recognize what I specifically needed and adapt to what science offered. Time was necessary for a cure and as I learned, time often seemed short, but it was it was important. I had to learn and accept that advice, professional and practical (what's necessary, not always the same). And I listened to those around me who cared — family, friends, peers. Remember,

peers are likely to be hypocritical and often, mine were. They disguised or otherwise didn't or wouldn't provide the honest and substantive guidance I desperately needed. So it became mandatory for loved-ones who were personally interested in my well-being to provide the basic guidance and advice. They may have suffered in the short run, putting up with my slowness of mind and body, my lack of mental ability, my shortness of temper, my mood swings, but they eventually won out and celebrated to see progress and results. And, I eventually recognized and accepted what they were doing. It must have been so difficult for them, so trying, but patience, understanding and love triumphed.

And I listened to me. At first life seemed threatening, overwhelming. Then through living that life, I realized that I had to put everything into perspective. Sure, there were problems, constantly, but I learned to accept that I'd been through something difficult. My survival brought with it both responsibility and reward, and it just seemed to be overwhelming. My responses were usually simple and usually not very adult-like. It was my "electrical system" that was affected and was malfunctioning and all previous experience was "shorted-out" and lost somewhere. While I had, have, other symptoms, other dilemmas, limitations, I am not an isolated being, but rather a piece of the puzzle of life and I found that by listening and seeing, I would soon become integrated in this great adventure of which I chose to still be a part.

✓ <u>PATIENCE</u>

Suffering without complaint is hard but most of the time I was successful. I tried to remember the old fable wherein patience led the turtle to victory over the hare. I had to rebuild old traits, make new ones. The damage to my mind seemed to highlight my ego to the point where it was no longer responsive to my will. It "ran" me. Stubbornness was constant, and it most often dominated. I presumed, and medicine concurred, that this happened because my body and mind were invaded and changed how both functioned. (To this day, put medication in my body and it affects my actions, my judgment, my speech.) Carelessness and irrational judgment and an overwhelming value of self also resulted. It was really that I was afraid, and it was the uncertainty that was disguising and mostly excusing my thoughts and actions — to me. As I look back, I am upset at the many false judgments based on emotionalism, not facts. But I also realized that it was part of my necessary growth. Fortunately, I had to face reality over and over, necessary for me to come out of all this mess, as good or better. As I look back at the "cure," those seemingly endless and elusive times, I can easily see the necessary "why'" — and I am reminded of that old project scheduling principle that says that the first 90 % of the project takes 90 % of the scheduled time — and the last 10 % takes the other 90 %. And, patience.

✓ WORK

I first thought that now was the chance to get away from it all — the pressure, the responsibility, the need to perform. But that couldn't happen. Reality came calling with just the opposite scenario. There was no job, not even a former life. The actions of others took it all away. I needed that part of my life to get better, a normal way of life, providing mental stimulation. Work would have assured those physical and mental demands that would make my body and my mind function. I could solve other problems rather than worry only about my own. My vocation, familiar surroundings, mental and physical stimuli would probably have stopped much of my floundering to regain a life lost. And I was lost. I needed all the help I could get. The ability and the opportunity to work provides an essential element that helps the mind and body regain much of what has been lost.

CHAPTER TWENTY-TWO
"Let Hertz Put You In The Driver's Seat"
(Hertz Corp., 1964)

It came to me one day that acceptance of this developing thing called a new me was going to depend a great deal on how I handled myself in regard to self-respect and self-confidence. Perhaps the most crushing and potentially destructive result of my stroke was a loss of both. I learned that it's often the case with a medical calamity when mental and physical abilities are upset and altered. Without these attributes to draw on when things got rough and tough, I just wouldn't be up to the challenge. Without these two attributes I couldn't be a constructive, productive person again.

✓ SELF-RESPECT
Self-respect is an essential element of a person's make up and as a contributing member of society. Without it, I stood naked, vulnerable and subject to the whims of others. So I had to rebuild, remodel and reload this most essential piece of me. Without respect for myself how could I expect to encourage respect from others? Regaining a` place in this world? The "pros" told me two things: it would never happen

or if I tried hard and I was lucky, well maybe. At least, in part. I felt obligated to give it a try because I was being given a second chance and I felt honor-bound to reward the torment , the suffering, the anxieties, the unselfishness offered me by my family and those few real friends (amazing, there were a few that stood by me.) And my mind kept repeating over and over: this is a great opportunity for me, to come to grips with myself, see and improve on what I am, what I can be, what I'm worth to myself and to others. And then there is the matter of self-respect's partner.

✓ SELF-CONFIDENCE

Self-confidence is best described as a state of feeling sure of the ability to be equal to anything demanded. Easy to say, harder to do. My initial actions appeared outwardly the opposite. My essential values were "missing in action." I was overly sensitive. I compensated by feigning false self-confidence, feigning strength of character and reliability to cover my actions of insecurity and bad judgment. Often having to face an inability to perform. Remember to listen. I couldn't tell by myself. And either I regained it or recovery was effectively stifled. By long trial and error, I found that only after regaining the self-confidence that was lost could I properly recognize and implement the necessary steps for my recovery. Lack of self-confidence coerced me into wallowing in self-pity, deceiving myself as to the true nature and extent of my progress and the ultimate goal. And without self-confidence I was ready to accept the mental and physical limitations imposed accepting most at face value. Not good enough. Not what could be. It was so shortsighted, yet, so simple to make excuses, so easy to accept the status quo — and easily settle for no improvement. Fortunately, with remonstrations and guidance from that angel of understanding who was my wife, my friend and partner in fortitude and confidence, I began to recognize the needed steps toward improvement. I rejoiced in the ever-growing feeling of success and the increasing ease of achieving. With self-confidence I looked more approvingly at that reflection in the mirror, smiled at the face that displayed the lines of life's battle, of defeat and victory, and the grey hair that life's experiences had awarded me. It was then that I knew that the ultimate battle was joined and that success could be the outcome. Doctors could note and pronounce that the physical body had improved about as far as it could go. The problem was now mental and most of that problem just might be repairable.

I sorely needed these two attributes because things were pretty rough. Medical insurance was cancelled. What insurance we could get for my wife and children cost a small fortune. Forget about me, I was rated (that means no insurance available). Living costs kept going up. We had to put food on the table and three children through school. High school was easy. College? Sacrifices were in order. My wife went back to work, took difficult, sometimes even menial jobs. Then better ones.. And, I had to face the real world, play the game, put it together, and get it together – again. I owed her. I owed my family. I owed myself.

It was an internationally known foundation with a half-century of good works (they were a client from my previous life). And the work was successful, a television series to millions of children and families weekly around the world. Then, running the whole operation — how lucky could I be. Looking back, I realize that those years were just practice, a "dry run" for the new challenges of how to be useful, to me, to others.

I now knew.

I hadn't "lost it."

I could do it.

The next opportunity was to travel and begin a new career - consulting. A crash course was necessary to get up to speed in a different world because I couldn't return to what had been. I had to put what little reputation I had on the line, teach people to be better at what they were doing and show them how it worked. Successful and effective, too (Yes, me with the "destroyed" brain — what was it now, about 10-12 years?)

Who says it can't come back.

We worked in teams, helped to correct the problems of dozens of ailing businesses, around the country. We taught retail businesses how to advertise accountably, knowing how much to spend and where and how to spend it. Then I studied and learned and subsequently implemented the essentials that made up successful enterprises. Of course, advertising and marketing I knew, but management, supervisory practice, financial, personnel (now

"H.R."), cost control, inventory, production, warehousing?

I gave seminars to hungry audiences and then worked with the people and businesses to make it happen. I gave speeches, made sales presentations and taught classes to the business personnel. Learning never really stops and with knowledge came self-respect and an ever-growing self-confidence. Experience really is the best teacher. And, yes, success helps. This confidence and newfound respect motivated me and my judgment and I remembered the truth in another old axiom: good judgment is the result of experience and experience is the result of bad judgment. Well, I had that going for me. There's a solution for everything, including me, and I grew bigger, stronger and better every time I faced and solved a problem. Then there were the foundations, the universities and fund-raising development. A whole new world was opening up.

It was all coming together.

And, it had better, for what was in store would present the greatest challenges of my life.

CHAPTER TWENTY-THREE
"Only Those Who Dare Truly Live"
(Ferrari, 1980)

Let's take stock. Was I ready to truly live? And, how?

While an impaired heart or kidney does not function or the cancer is bad and might spread elsewhere, arteries remain clogged or restricted, whatever the prognosis, time is on your side and time has a unique way of healing, if you give it a chance.

Sure, it took a long time, but medicine is so improved. I am not a "vegetable." I am not seriously mentally or physically impaired. Today, I give every appearance of being a normal, healthy person and it's been a long "practice run." The years of this confinement of mind and body taught me more than a man has a right. I learned knowledge and wisdom and how to prosper because of it. I learned, and I think I know, what this world, what we are about. I learned how to get to the root of things, to be a necessary part. I forced myself to take positions and make a stand for what I now knew was right. Organization and direction are essential because confusion is the worst of all possible solutions to nothing.

I didn't do it alone. Someone had to recognize who I was, what I was and what I was doing — family, friends, business associates. Remember, family is emotionally involved. Family will often overlook or downplay mistakes, ignore obvious problems, excuse behavior because it was "just a bad day," or believe that it will all go away and wasn't really that serious. Wrong, because it all leads to their giving and you taking.

I did it. It's the easy way. And friends have their own problems, and as much as they may want to help, they first have to "till their own garden."

It may take time, hopefully not too much, but business associates' input is invaluable because it's timely and fact-based and usually unbiased. Through them, you are forced to see the facts and the hard truth, to make choices and not just live securely (but unhappily) in an ineffective, non-productive world of make-believe. It all began to make sense, experience (that 90 % - 90 % axiom) began to tell me what was right or wrong and if I'd done the proper homework Life. Adapt and cope. It's part of winning or losing. In my beginnings, more of the latter — but then the former started to come and more and more easily. I got serious about life.

And I had to ask myself some hard questions:
- ✓ *Am I happy being what I am?*
- ✓ *Was it better than not being counted at all?*
- ✓ *Am I doing things capably?*
- ✓ *Do I work for "complete" recovery (what is "complete?") or would I rather stay like*

I am? Because it's comfortable?
- ✓ *So I'm not really happy, all the way. Is that a crime? I'm pretty good.*
- ✓ *And it's so warm and safe in here. Let someone else make the choices, save the world. I've been through so much already, why more?*

And these were the answers:
- ✓ *I'm not just the same. I'm a better person.*
- ✓ *I am more responsive and more productive.*
- ✓ *I have stronger and more selective values.*
- ✓ *I can accomplish things, better things and more of them.*
- ✓ *If I'm not where I want to be yet, I will be.*
- ✓ *Stop thinking and just DO!*

And more. Think of where you've been and what you've become.

The big question is really quite simple: What do you do with this recovery and that is the ultimate test of your new life. It is time to take all that has happened, all the positive, life-affirming, thankful-to-be-granted-a-second-chance energy and put it to good use.

It was time to make a difference

CHAPTER TWENTY-FOUR
"Got Milk"
(California Milk Processing Board, 1993)

Snoopy, that talented beagle in the "Peanuts" comic strip, always begins his story: "it had been a very dark and stormy night". Well, it had been. Rain had kept the land company all the night before and that land was now an endless expanse of dirty-gray-brown soup stretching from eye to horizon, an endless sea of waste broken at times with small craggy-looking and drab greenery and constructions of some sort that once were landscaped farms and cultivated land where people had dwelled and toiled. It used to be called civilization. It was now better described as desolation. This was the disaster flood, appropriately named the "Midwet," as the Mississippi and Missouri Rivers and many other smaller waterways overflowed some seven Midwestern states. Cities, land, people — there were no exceptions. It was big. It was a big mess. The year was 1993.

Sure, It had been some years now but contrary to accepted prognosis, I had actually progressed enough through this "terminal illness and disability," through consulting, thinking again and the other work accomplishment to put all the new-found and old experience and learning to work on a bigger stage. I was still doing all that I had learned, able to do it on my own now, but found that I needed regularity, support and a bigger stage. It was a very important "stage" as I was to find out. It was the Federal Emergency Management Agency. FEMA, as it is more commonly known, helps others to regain lost lives and property and face down the apocalypses called flood, earthquake, hurricane, tornado and fire.

Impossible, you ask? No. Responsibility, sureness, effectiveness, worth were now in my grasp. I couldn't waste what I had been through and learned. I was taking charge of my life again, visualizing the outcome, planning and acting accordingly.

Yes, life was beginning again and it was time for that difference.

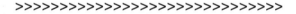

Morning rubbed its eyes. The skies were still overcast, the weather all one color — gloom. Clouds peered through other clouds. More of the wet stuff was forecast. The mood of headquarters pretty much matched the weather when I arrived for work just as daylight was beginning. One could just feel that it was going to be "that kind of day..."

My piece of the puzzle started with public information and the media. The job was to put a positive face on the disaster, the hard work, the successes, the setbacks, the people. But, as we'll see, knowledge and experience usually led to other chores, from field work with disaster victims to "trouble-shooting" other damage problems and controls. In this instance, having had prior experience with animal welfare matters, I was urgently called upon by a concerned Humane Society of the United States (HSUS). I had a long working relationship with that organization. There were twenty-five head of cattle stranded on a piece of land surrounded by rapidly rising waters. Try to picture these frightened animals huddled and muddled and milling around. Everyone was concerned as reports indicated that these cattle would soon be swallowed by the unstoppable onslaught of water. Something had to be done. And, now!

"Hello, Coast Guard? This is FEMA, St. Louis. This is an emergency and we need your help. May I speak with someone in charge of disaster matters?" Hopefully, my words conveyed a feeling of urgency, because the person at the other end of the line seemed to be in the same mood as the weather. .

After some switching, and the usual dead time, I managed to speak with someone of authority, one who professed professionalism and seemed to know something and perhaps could do something.

"I realize that you're probably "snowed under" and your resources are stretched pretty thin. That goes for all of us, doesn't it? But, we've got an immediate and unusual problem and really need your help. There are 25 head of cattle isolated on a piece of land over near the airport in Bainbridge, and it's going to be flooded over and those cattle are all going to drown. They can't swim in this stuff, all the mess. I know that these aren't people, but they have a right to live, too. Besides, they're worth a lot of money and we're going to need all we can get to make this country well again."

The conversation continued a bit, and then:

"I can have what? A rowboat?" I incredulously questioned. "To move 25 head of cattle? They're too big and even if we could, with a dozen trips minimum, there wouldn't be enough time — the land will be gone and so will the cattle."

Then an idea began.

"This rowboat — is it big enough to hold four-five people?"

"Yes," came the answer.

"OK," I replied. "Would you fill it with life preservers and lots of rope and meet us in, say, about an hour where the Mississippi makes a big bend just before Bainbridge, underneath the schoolhouse on the bluff?"

A plan was taking shape. Maybe there was hope yet — for the cows, and for me.

I hung up, keeping a short fuse on a shorter leash and only thinking that I just couldn't imagine such shortsightedness, much less, stupidity.

The next step was HSUS.

"Can you meet me with four or five bodies at the schoolhouse over near Bainbridge. You know, the one on that big bluff overlooking the Mississippi where those cattle are stranded. I've got a plan that should work. I'll get there as fast as these flooded roads will allow. Give me about 45 minutes."

I couldn't drive yet and besides, another body

could help. Marty got the job. He knew. He'd help. And, we drove as fast as safe, splashing showers and waves in our wake, swerving to avoid downed trees and other of nature's obstacles (glad no one was with us, no grab-bars in this car). I prayed some that there'd be enough time. And I rehearsed it over in my mind. It made sense but its execution was something else. I should also have wondered about me, for my physical abilities were not yet much at this stage of recovery and just what help could I offer? But adrenalin got in the way and I didn't think that far ahead. Just get there and do!

It was mid-morning by the time we reached the Schoolhouse. HSUS was there with four people, John, Paul, Steve and Kathy, to face an inflated, roiling and dirty waterway. We were six and the Coast Guard was down there somewhere to help. As we hiked down, I explained the plan, and hoped.

"We make a raft with tree trunks and any suitable logs and tie them to the life preservers. The Coast Guard has enough of all this stuff with them in the boat and then we just float the cattle of." It sounded so efficient and simple.

We finally arrived at the river, saw the Coast Guard and the boat - with a sinking feeling. In unison, Kathy and Steve cried out, "Those aren't life PRESERVERS, they're life JACKETS!" In a disgusted voice, John added, "Those animals will sink like a rock in this stuff!"

Ever the optimist, I tried to be diplomatic: "Let's take what we've got and give it a try."

In all the confusion, the Coast Guard hastily disappeared. I had counted on their help.

Hope was wearing thin. But we began. (It might be a fruitless endeavor, but like this whole book, you've got to try, no matter the odds. And in some way, some form, you'll succeed.)

It took a while and all that while we kept glancing at the rising water, hoping against hope. The odds were not on our side. We tried to make do. We made the logs and gathered the wood. We tied the life jackets to the bottom and we forged a "makeshift" vessel, a sort of raft and when it looked sturdy enough, Paul jumped aboard and cast off. It floated! There was hope!

"Hot damn," he spouted. And we cajoled and prodded and luckily herded all the frightened cattle onto our "vessel."

It promptly sank.

And we now had the problem of swimming out in that mess and rescuing twenty-five head of very frightened, confused and skittish animals from themselves.

So much for Plan One. Field conditions required an Alternate Plan Two.

The angry river was just too deep, too fast and filled with passing trees and brush and garbage to attempt a fording. And on foot we could do little if anything in guiding these cattle to safety. So there was only one thing left to do if we were going to have a rescue at all.

"We've got life jackets. Why wouldn't they work on the animals and then we might be able to make it across the river just like in those old days." I couldn't give up. Any port in a storm, as they say, or maybe I'd watched too many Westerns.

But we had to at least try. We, I'd, come this far. Maybe there was a way.

We all took turns at being "wranglers." Couldn't the cattle tell that we were just trying to help them?

Picture. Six adult humans trying to fit a rather small life harness onto an animal that probably thought we were either trying to inflict harm or were just plain stupid for trying something that the animal knew all along wouldn't work. There was a very frightened black and white with a somewhat glazed look that might have been affection or even understanding. So, I thought, let's try her first. I moved to put a life jacket over her head. Bad choice. Affection or even understanding turned to fear and panic. Her eyes flashed and she flashed and snorted and lashed, kicked up and out, knocking me into the lovely water. You'd have thought she was a Brahma Bull in a rodeo. Good facsimile. Me? I looked the clown, dripping wet and all dirty to boot.

All tried their hand. Similar results.

Marty said, "Let me, I've got an idea." He corralled another cow, got her close to the water, but it was he who took the bath.

We all tried. Picture a scene of complete bedlam, six fairly rugged humans trying to put a life preserver over the head, around the neck, the fore legs, the hind legs, blindfolding the animal first. Whatever the way, the cattle all remained dry, and we were the ones that ended with the problems. The kicking and snorting and bucking cows managed to knock most of us into those soupy, smelly waters, leaving cuts and bruises behind. We all looked as if we had been in a barroom brawl.

Enough for "brilliant" Plan Two.

Finally, with help from some socially-conscious people back at the DAC, we managed to rent a barge, towed it to that little (and getting smaller by the moment) piece of land and got all the cattle off — in time!

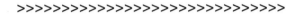

>>>>>>>>>>>>>>>>>>>>>>>>>>>>>>>>>>>>

After all this, I was determined that such misunderstandings, such callous attitudes toward another part of the animal world should never happen again. It took a lot of work, travel and talk, seminars and socializing, posturing and politicking, three years, another three disasters and the aid of some other concerned people and organizations to cut through a lot of red tape, hurting a lot of feelings and bruising many an ego. Washington, D.C. may be a tough town, but those in government finally realized that rescuing livestock and companion animals in emergency situations should be a priority, just like it is for us, people. It's in writing and in the Directives. The media has recognized the wide appeal of the matter and is helping spread the word.

I don't work for FEMA anymore, but my legacy does.

CHAPTER TWENTY-FIVE
"Will Miracles Never Cease?"
(Xerox, 1977)

So much for the physical, was the mind up to the task? Was my "revamped" mind ready to make that difference?

They brought him into the room, to face the desk. He was of medium build and height. He was cuffed at the wrists, with manacles on his feet. The police hovered over his every movement. His clothes were dirty and torn, almost hanging on a spare frame, clothes that were once expensive in tailoring and fabric were now reduced to benefit shop rags. Strange, for one slovenly of appearance, unshaven, hair tousled and matted, just like a street person. And his eyes, cold and penetrating, loudly pronounced his hatred for everyone and everything.

In those earlier days disaster relief was not organized by a computer in a sterile central location, away for all harm. There were Disaster Assistance Centers (called DACs) set-up in each city affected by any disaster. They were usually located in schools because these complexes offered an auditorium or gymnasium for maximum usable space and were normally built on high ground. All disaster-related services were represented at desks (with plenty of chairs) around the perimeter of the room — Salvation Army, Red Cross, Small Business Association, local banks, attorneys, construction firms, hospitals, care, rescue facilities, appropriate businesses and people would efficiently go from desk to desk to solve their problems with whatever restraint and dignity they had left. It was the personal touch, and it worked well.

However, every once in a while, there was a glitch.

The man had reluctantly slouched in the chair opposite. He acknowledged my presence with a curt nod and almost a grunt. I shuffled through the material in front of me, hopefully looking nonchalant and attempting to appear concerned. I was shaken but curious.

"What's your name?" I queried.

"Mark," he replied, then grudgingly added, "Twain."

My surprise was obvious, so I half-jokingly asked, "From where?"

His reply was just as surprising, "Hannibal, up river."

I looked more closely at the man. This was going to be difficult, at best. I asked myself, is he kidding me — same name, same place?

"Where in Hannibal?" I asked, forcing concern into my voice. Then, without waiting for a reply, I plunged ahead.

"You don't exactly look and act like a man who should be handcuffed and locked away. I'd like to try to help. There's a problem here and I hope you can give me some answers, information to go on."

I was trying to convince myself, to buy in to this man's problems because there was something very wrong here, his carriage, his manner, his dress — it just didn't add up.

The man's visage remained passive, face rigid, as if of sterner stuff. But I glimpsed a fleeting trace of response, even hope in his eyes, then a slight relaxing of the facial muscles. One learns to "read people" in this job.

"The first thing we do is get rid of those cuffs and shackles — now, has anyone you talked with really listened?"

Suddenly, the wall came down. As the metal restraints were taken off, a torrent of words came out in broken, often halting fashion,

"I tried to get help. I went to your center at the middle school three times. And they started in again, giving me the run-around. So I said I'd better get some action this time or I'd start shooting. I don't know with what because I didn't even start to have a weapon anymore. But I said that I was tired of waiting. My home, my land was under tons 'o water, my livestock had just about all drowned, no clothes, no money, no nothing, and then they shot my dog and tried to rape my wife. How much is a man supposed to take? And I pleaded, who gives out the help? Who'd I have to see?

"Then this man comes over, grabs a hold of me and shouts, 'Get out of here before I call the police! That did it. I don't look very nice, the muddy waters and life took care of that. But police? I was stupid. I grabbed back and shook him. Everyone ran. Bedlam. And here I am, assault, battery, attempted bodily harm —

it goes on. They ran drug tests, put me in a solitary cell. Hell, I have a name. I'm a person, not a number. But it seems that nobody knows who or what I am, what I need. Or, really gives a damn."

He ran out of breath, and anger.

"I don't know all the answers, but we'll find them," I said, responding to all this, a bit angry now, too, and more than a bit perplexed but no longer hesitant or confused.

"I'm no attorney, but there has to be a way to straighten out this mess. And, you're no criminal. Tell me more," I urged. "It seems rather stupid and shortsighted just ignore your problems and what you need, treat you badly, try to do things like the rules say. Sometimes, one has to bend a few and answer some hard questions about those rules."

Suffice it to say that this story had a happy ending as did so many more like it from so many other disasters. Yes, he was released, to resume a full and contributory life in his world. Importantly, the fact of my functioning again, better, is best summed–up in the comments innocently made to Mark Twain that day:

"Hang in there, my friend. Your namesake had his ups and downs. But, he ended up a winner. You will, too. You just need a small miracle. I had a miracle once. Let's see if I can turn one for you."

CHAPTER TWENTY-SIX
"You're In Good Hands"
(Allstate Insurance, 1950)

Not necessarily in this order, but the three most appropriate words to describe my continued existence on this planet are God, guts and my wife. It took all three to make me into a whole. I'm a married man, and so the reference – it could also be husband, significant other, partner, whatever fits. Guts leads to a few thoughts on courage and belief in myself and maybe more. God? Another name might do. It's all a part of religion and it's a very personal matter. That's why these next passages were so difficult. It's hard enough to explain, much less put into words and on paper. It has to do with the soul, the inner being that we've all got. As long as it serves to help, what do names matter? Know that it's well worth it. Nothing is hopeless. If you try, you can work miracles.

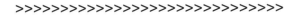

I'm not the most devout person. But I am spiritual and have some religion and belief. Most people do, in some fashion, whether they recognize it as such or not. We don't live alone with just pride and faith in ourselves, believing that fate and fortune will carry us. Especially not with this, my situation. God, or whatever name one uses, will collect his due when it suits the purpose, and since this Almighty gave us brains and a free will, tested by the eons of practice and error, doesn't it logically follow that we are the means, the tools, to work in the desired way, until that time? Or, if one believes only in the theory of scientific evolution and disavows the existence of a supreme being, then think about it this way: We grew from an amoeba or a fish or an ape. We struggled onto land from the sea or stood upright or ran or hunted or painted pictures or made noises (like my earlier days). But there was always something that acted as a catalyst, that made it happen, that controlled the process and orderly growth (the world has never been disorderly, either in its formation or action.) Fish can't write, apes can't write, but man can and did when he put down what he believed and that's where religion came from and by the grace of something or someone's control, so did you and I. Whether male or female is unimportant to the point — I'm being generic. Don't dismiss this out of hand, this is all leading to somewhere important.

Paul, while lecturing in Athens those many centuries ago, was right on target when he spoke of an unknown God, a supreme and all-knowing being. Either you believe or you don't. It is not something that you can rationally explain. Belief may be in this supreme being, your fellow creatures, the trees, the stars, the state, even yourself. But my adventure should prove to you that mankind is not strong enough, alone. One must rely upon something else, stronger, better, to see it through. Life was, is too complex, too sophisticated to accept the principles and mores of our ancestors at face value. You've got to consider your values, your needs, now and for the future. That's why this tale, why the admonitions and the guides.

Let's go back to what happens with a stroke (or a heart attack, a trauma, an injury, a cancer or whatever serious illness or operation).

What happens to the body? What happens to the mind? Is it just a painful and excusable malady? Are there fantasies? What does all this have to do with religion? I had to answer these questions based on the need to satisfy, to justify my own continued existence. Who else can be as objective and honest with themselves? Rationalize? Not the typical, making excuses. Rather, rationalize in the sense of making something more comfortable ("rationalize" as being reasonable in ordinary and normal thought). Yes, that was finally beginning to come around some. But I also found that faith in one's self just wasn't enough. It didn't, couldn't do the job by itself. Is this proof? Part. You've got to have a belief to come through whatever. But if that's all, who's to tell if it's right or wrong? I had to come up with my own solution, something that satisfied me. And, I did. When I needed it, the strength was forthcoming.

There were two important happenings that transpired during my illness and rehabilitation. Agree with the following or not, the facts stand and it all happened as described. You be the judge.

When the calamity, the cerebral hemorrhage hit, I was paralyzed, a vegetable not long for this world. I don't remember the ambulance, the hospital, or the people who helped. But to this day there is one clear recollection. A tunnel, a very long and very black tunnel, and I was going through that tunnel. There was a light at the end of that tunnel. I never reached the end but my light was certainly "turned on." There was no fanfare, no pretty music. But the episode tells that the teachings and accounts of religion are true: when a person has a near death or death experience, there is a tunnel and a light at the end and the light represents the ultimate salvation in life. Mine, as it turned out, and this story relates the result.

The second instance occurred when faith in myself, my faith in a higher being, anything, was stretched pretty thin. I was desolate; I was disconsolate; I was beside myself with self-pity and reproach about progress that just wasn't. My reactions were slow. In my tepid mental state at that time I guess it was just give-in and take the easy way out of it all. It was only about six weeks after experiencing my fate, and I was in the second of those hospitals. And, one night, in my sleep, I almost expired, "bought it", died. Then there was a dream and a deep and commanding voice in that dream said to me that life was really worth living and if it's worth living then it was worth fighting for, that there was much good in life and only by living could I be a part.

Whose voice doesn't matter because this whole story tells the "who", I knew and we now all know.

From that night to this day, I've had other visits and dreams, some strong guidance and very sound advice. Again and again. I've made mistakes, but I've grown and progressed from them. I take pride in the accomplishments and looking back, know that these years were a practice for that which I was promised, for becoming a new and better person — the experiences, the growing, the challenges of how to be of use, met and conquered. There were "down" times, there were "up" times

But there were always "can do" times. That's why this book. I tried. I like the result.

Both my wife and I have been granted the strength and patience to have made it to today. Say it was "guts," you're right. Say it was my "wife," my friend and companion in life, you're right. One cannot come through all this without help from both within and without. Say it was "God," you're right. There are things in religion that I have found wanting, but the principles are there for a good reason. I accepted them at face value and then decided what was right for me. That's what being here is all about. Otherwise there are going to be insurmountable problems and unnecessary anguish — and recovery just isn't going to happen.

CHAPTER TWENTY-SEVEN
"Have It Your Way"
(Burger King Restaurants, 1974)

Since we're analyzing things that affect survival and recovery, how about the role of medicine and hospitals?

Much time has passed. Much life has passed. A better life, a very productive life is my good fortune. Medicine has also come a long way. There are now anti-coagulants, beta/channel blockers, pacemakers, tools and drugs to pull out or dissolve clots from arteries to stop strokes, the list goes on. Radiation, chemotherapy, angioplasty, have all been improved and are not nearly so invasive or painful. Magnetic Reasoning (MRIs), CT Scans, PET Scans, other tests can now pinpoint problems so that the doctors can isolate the distressed areas, take computer pictures to vertically and horizontally dissect and analyze problems for their correction. Today, one is in and out of the hospital in a shorter time, in and out of illness in a shorter time.

My doctor and friend, Cy, our wives and I were discussing illness and recovery some time after the hospitals and my struggles toward health and wellness. It was a fine visit over a hearty lunch and a good reminiscence of what was. Cy started it all with an answer to my continuing questions.

"Remember, Dick, it's really up to you, the patient, to tell all to the physician so that he or she can make the right diagnosis and decisions. Doctors are human, too, and we can make mistakes. We just know more because we've studied the specifics and got to practice our craft."

"With a lot of sacrifice," Shirley, Cy's wife, admonished.

"OK," I commented, "I think I did my part and you did yours. We're both still here and better people. But how could I have avoided all the hassle? It's been a very long time and it was a bit hard to take – for me, for anyone."

Cy's response? "You had a wake-up call, to a longer and better life. They just weren't ready for you yet, your number wasn't called, as they say. First, lifestyle choices are necessary, now and before it all happened. Remember, I tried to get you to change, but you were so stubborn.

"Amen, to that," interjected Nancy.

"You did exercise, and you stopped smoking, I'll hand that to you," proclaimed the good doctor. "And, you stay in good shape." (For the shape I'm in, I thought to myself.)

Nancy again entered the fray. "But your diet stinks, eating all that cholesterol and carbohydrates. I can't eat it. Why should you? You've got to change, and I'll help."

"And there's stress, every-day fatigue and we all know that the psychological demands of life work subtly on the ways we think and feel.

So we have to stack the deck in our favor

whenever we can — that's where my husband's insistence on diet and good health comes in," added Shirley.

"If nothing else, I've learned two important things," I stated. "You've got to take control over your life. We can't face the world's problems alone, can't control the events, but we can control how we react to them and handle them. And, we decide the what and the where and handle those problems based on our knowledge and experience, input from others and just plain common sense that life's experiences have taught us."

"And," pronounced my wife, "you've got to be positive, network with us, your family, and with your friends. Unwind with relaxation whenever there's a chance, reading, music, games, even work around the house, inside and out — those 'honey-dos' you love so much."

I've always wondered," queried Shirley, "there must be similarities between what Dick had and other calamities of life. What do you do then, dear?"

"Let me answer this way." Cy spoke with the authority of the administrator of the hospital where it had all started, "Getting well is more than just having the pain go away and your life and energy level getting back to normal. There are medical and psychological problems associated with any illness, any surgery, any hospitalization. It all depends on what, cancer, heart, vascular, stroke. The patient may face delirium, anxiety in fear of the unknown and the uncertainty of the future. There may even be denial, not wanting to face reality, the facts, and the patient may well exhibit behavioral problems, like not cooperating with the caregivers, not adjusting to this new situation.

"Then the patient may exhibit what we call 'ICU Psychosis' which entails sleep deprivation, social isolationism, perhaps even delirium. And when the patient gets out of ICU and back to a halfway reasonable existence in the hospital with care and supervision, the patient may then have guilt, or an attempt to escape reality, even a masochistic need to suffer. Then we have to face the patient-family syndrome: the patient, the family, are overly demanding and there may be disputes with the staff, often accompanied by infantile behavior. There may even be sexual advances to the doctor or nurse. The patient is frustrated and this is a way of 'reaching out.' To solve such problems there's got to be one head, one person that the patient can trust and that individual can oversee multiple treatments, solve multiple problems. Our life isn't that easy either."

"Wow! That's a mouthful to digest, along with this great food. I wasn't a model patient and I guess I did some of all that. Don't remember any sex, though," I turned to my wife with a twinkle in my eye, "Must have been too weak and mentally messed up. Seriously, what about the long recuperation period after the hospital ?" I questioned.

Cy responded with his usual wisdom, "The key here is patience and understanding. The patient has got to get involved with life through society first. You've worked with service, support organizations. Forgive the philosophy, but charitable work comes next because it provides accomplishment and a rush of adrenalin called success, then business in whatever. One knows when he or she is ready."

"And don't forget the support areas," Nancy professionally added, she being a former teacher and community leader, "other people, the internet, the library. Knowledge about the disease is so very helpful in setting the right mental attitude, before, during and after. There wasn't anything available about what you had, Dick, all they could do was refer to it as a 'seizure' or 'apoplexy'. There needs to be something and someone so that you can understand what is, what happens, what's expected. It would have helped me to comprehend and cope with it, and you."

I thought: *And, there is a need for something else.*

CHAPTER TWENTY-EIGHT
"Leave The Driving To Us"
(Greyhound Lines, 1956)

Laughter and a sense of humor is an important, an almost essential part of the healing process. It does wonders for getting rid of those mental barriers and problems. So far in my new life, and to this point in the story, everything had been pretty serious and very probably because it's a serious matter. However, laughing at and with life proved a necessary part of recovery and rejuvenation..

Not much to laugh about in those early days. Humor seemed immaterial. But I can now look back with a wry chuckle at those often absurd occurrences, happenings in a gradually broadening life, adventures that transpired, standing out as examples of stubbornness,

even stupidity, yet all necessary to recovery and reasserting my place in this world. When I think of what might have been or might have happened. It's so important to laugh at yourself, at the world, and learn from it.

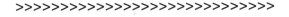

I had driven an automobile just once since my stroke. Early on, maybe three years after it happened. It was a test lap around that lake by our home. The scenery added a touch of romance and elegance to the exercise. My wife accompanied and played instructor. The big vehicle, a safe and family-sized car, a station wagon that was the standard for family vehicles in that time - SUVs were still simply Jeeps from WWII and back roads were far from my needs. And that smaller, ego-machine with a stick shift that complemented my earlier life, demanded coordination between hand and eye, muscle and mind, and that I couldn't produce. The trip went well, or at least I thought so (shall we call it a grand experiment) and later, Nancy confessed that she had girded herself with prayer and tranquilizers prior to the adventure. Yes, it was an adventure.

The next step seemed relatively simple — for me. It was some time later and it involved driving my oldest daughter to a school function.

"Are you sure you should do this, Dad? Really, I think that my friends can drive me. Dad, that's really a funny way of getting in the car.

"That's not the way Mom holds that wheel. Dad, I'm scared!" — Lisa was thinking it best to get out of the car but I had pressed the lock button and she was trapped.

"Don't you worry, young lady, I know what I'm doing, been making these things perform for more years than you are. You're in safe hands." I postulated this in a somewhat slurred fashion, heartfelt but not nearly good enough to instill confidence in my young daughter.

The master of the byways calmly began to move the vehicle. "Just sit tight, young lady, everything's fine, Dad knows just what he's doing."

My daughter sat beside me, mostly paralyzed with fear, unable to comment, as I meandered down the road. (It was mostly straight, only those "autocross-type" curves that seemed to appear at odd times. They seemed like the corkscrew turns at a raceway, but we're getting ahead of things, for I didn't know about raceways, then).

"See how we make all these turns, so gracefully." (someone upstairs was looking after me – or rather, her) At least I wasn't driving on the wrong side of the road, just down the middle, recovering to the right from time to time.

"Watch out for that poor lady," rousing from her paralysis, my daughter yelled in horror, and I swerved in time.. *Obviously it was her fault*, I thought.

We fortuitously arrived at our destination. My daughter was understandably upset but retained her outward demeanor of confidence. She was not an overly religious child but I'm sure that she prayed a lot, that we'd arrive sooner than soon.

"We're here, Dad, please, can I get out and walk with… Oh, there's my good friend, Judie..." She pushed open the door and jumped out without waiting for further instruction.

"Meet you inside," she shouted over her shoulder, with relief all over her voice as she flew into a crowd of young people.

The destination was only a short way from home (otherwise I may not have been allowed) and was appropriately a school traffic affair where young people learn responsibility for school safety crossings, speed limits, stop signs and all that. Perhaps I was learning, too.

There were many friends and acquaintances, all astounded to see me and initially groping for the right things to say, bending over backwards to be sociable and polite.

My comments were loud and repetitive. My daughter wasn't just embarrassed, she was mortified, trying desperately to melt into the woodwork. Her jovial and proud but very stupid parent tried to chat with everyone. (You have to try.)

"Great food, grand affair, good friends, good to see you, good to be here," my words were slurred over and over and over again. Commenting further with an extended vocabulary: "This is wild" (everything was "wild," I'm told) and "This is my lovely and talented oldest daughter."

Ad nauseam.

After the repast and the usual speaker, the dreaded return drive was in the offing. If only my daughter had been older, she could have driven the return trip with more accuracy than I. That we arrived home safely is attested to by this book and my daughter's happy and productive life. Small wonder, however, she became a psychology major in college and still has reservations about my driving ability.

But there is more to it than "chuckles."

CHAPTER TWENTY-NINE
"Just Do It!"
(Nike, 1988)

They say laugh and the world laughs with you. I badly needed to rediscover my sense of humor, relearn to laugh. To date there hadn't been much, outside of laughing at myself. But this was all a worthwhile struggle with a happy ending, because I faced the matter squarely and took the problems seriously and always searched for a way to find the humor in the situation. These small examples tell and hopefully, demonstrate. Simply, it was the concept of looking at matters objectively and laughing at them, and at myself. It was an essential element to my satisfactory recovery. In a simpler sense, I learned to recognize that the problems, the challenges, were really just pieces of life that had to be met and resolved and remembering that humor and laughter were a necessary part.

To recap:" the medics had given up on any physical ability. Muscle control and motor functions were destroyed, some temporarily, others forever. Indoor activities such as squash and handball were out. Table tennis was for the Olympics, not me. Card games required concentration, memory, analysis and I didn't have them. Team sports? I was too old.

Individual outdoor sports, forget it. Accepted medical dogma said that I'd never again play any sport, much less one which required any form of balance and coordination. But, as the lyricist, Gilbert astutely wrote: "Well, hardly ever."

I had to start somewhere. I thought I was ready. But someone forgot to tell the rest of the world.

Initial excursions into physical activity occurred with my son (poor guy). First there was baseball. It started with playing catch, fortunately with mitts — my attempting to throw straight and he, valiantly trying to catch the ball, high, low, way-y-y-y outside. Wild pitches were commonplace, the strike zone almost invisible to me. My wife, a good ballplayer, and daughters all needed to keep a straight face. Then "catch" graduated to every father's duty of Little League. I tried desperately to walk straight, talk straight. Embarrassment must have been difficult for my son to endure. But I guess that just my being there meant something. From baseball we graduated to football. Throwing presented the same problem. Small wonder he grew to be good — eventually, a good coach and a good teacher.

Camping and fishing were next on the list, my son, the "guinea pig." Picture the scene: the formerly proficient fisherman, staggering against the current, legs and arms not coordinating, attempting to cast a line and catch a fighting fish while standing in the middle of the roiling waters of a healthy river. I was rather wet when I struggled to shore to quickly start a fast-drying campfire. One can't eat clothes, but dry ones work better for cooking the real stuff. And after such exercise, sleeping was never a problem for me, though I'm sure that my son may have had some sleepless nights.

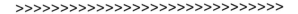

After many years of recuperative existence and hiding behind the familiar in the San Francisco area, traveling, growing, testing the waters, we ventured south to the Monterey Peninsula and a new life. This next step in my "rehabilitation" became obvious (besides, wasn't this the golfing "mecca" of the West?) Besides, golf has a handicap. And golf has many similarities to life. It's fun and stimulating and it's a chance to compete against yourself and nature.

But, I'd never played golf before. A challenge?

Balance and coordination, well, I'd have to learn, or at least, try. It meant a lot of time (I had that) and practice, practice, practice. Teaching the motor functions how to do what the mind thought and communicated was not easy. There were times when I felt, that nothing like this activity could work. Then there were times when I was beside myself with joy at being able to do something well. I had to prepare for the good days and bad. The medical people had said I couldn't do it and gave me all the reasons and golfers just threw up their hands. And, I just looked at it all like the game of life and "went for it," having learned that life, too, is hard work and it, too, had rules and rewards. You always feel better when you work toward a solution.

That first time was a true disaster: slicing to the right, hooking to the left, readily finding trees, sand, water and other obstacles (when I managed to hit the ball.) Putting was easier - just point, push and pray. I thought. I guess ignorance is bliss. Hopefully a lesson or two would help.

"Now you hold the club loosely but firmly, thus," the "pro" admonished. "No, not with a death grip. Hands like this. Fingers hold the club. Let it rest in your hands — thus. Imagine you're holding a bird in your hands, too loose, he'll fly away, too tight and you'll crush him. Form a 'V' with your thumb and first finger. Now, with the other hand, line up the 'Vs — thus.

"Now, just watch me. This is how your swing should be. Plant your feet about shoulder width, stand about this far back from the ball, about the club length, making sure that your arms are loose, the ball should be just inside your left foot, and the left elbow pointed toward the left hip, right arm loose, left arm straight as you take the back swing, and make sure that your hands at the top of the swing are high and the shaft points along a line parallel to the ground and when you swing through remember that the weight is 60 per cent on the left foot and 40 per cent on the right and as you come through you turn the right knee in toward the left as the right heel comes off the ground and make sure that the hands turn over the left foot as you turn and follow through — except when you're hitting on the fairway, when the ball is between your feet or pitching or chipping, and then the feet are moved this way and the ball is positioned differently, back in your stance, weight on our left foot, but then you must move it and aim left or right on uphill or downhill lies, and different when you get caught in the "bunker," and then you anchor your feet with weight on the back foot and take a full swing and when you putt you stand thusly and make a full and easy straight swing, keeping the arms straight, your hands are a hinge, head down, etc., etc., etc. ... remember to swing easy and keep your head down and still at all times because if you move it you're screwed and you'll have to start all over again. Now, you try."

This guy just didn't realize that I couldn't do it that way. But the basics are the basics and you do it right, follow the rules, use a little reason or don't even try. And I thought to myself as I tried:

Words. Actions. How did I come to deserve all of this? How am I going to remember all this? Maybe, over time? Sounds like all the doctors' rules, and life's rules. Well, better safe than sorry. Damn the trajectory, I don't care where, how far, if I can just manage to hit that damn little white thing. How can I possibly "coordinate" in my condition. No excuses. Just do it!

Picture, if you will, the amateur "chump," dressed the part according to the magazines and the images on television, tense and up-tight, the very picture of a stressed-out person, attacking that tiny white sphere. The wood club is raised, poised, forced downward toward the small white ball and with a mighty stroke that would send that ball hundreds of yards down that stretch of immense and gorgeous green grass. "Swoosh" — and the club rent the air and missed the ball. It was a real-life "Casey at the Bat" and the air was shattered with the force of the blow.

To make a long story short, with the patience of a good teacher and my money on the line, the "pro" began anew. He showed me the foibles of my efforts and the error of my ways. He observed and commented as I did it again and again and again and again.

"See, practice makes perfect," he said, handing me the rest of the iggest bucket of balls I'd ever seen. "Just go to that range over there and hit the rest of these balls."

It was a long day, an exhausting day, but I instinctively felt that this day marked a new beginning of a really satisfying life. Sure it was frustrating, but it was also so worth it. It's all in how you look at it, handle it. You really are happier when you work for a solution.

Since that first time, things have improved. Yes, golf is a challenge mentally, physically, and when you're on your game, short or long or both, it's really worth it. Like life, itself. When I overdo it takes a good while for the "electrical system" and the coordination and balance to return. Like life, there are good days and bad. Like life, there are good times and bad. And like life, there are good friends and bad. But on the golf course, there are mostly good friends who help and understand. And teach because of it.

There were many, many more things in my

experiences, my growing pains, to laugh at, to laugh with, to laugh about. Compensating and learning. Growth feeds on itself to push for bigger and better results. Complacency is only an invitation to a lessened recovery and a less rewarding existence. I could laugh at myself, again, and with the world. Oh, I made plenty of excuses, really trying to rationalize — more to myself than anyone else. There's still a need. But that's my problem. The golf course is a special, fun place for camaraderie and friendship and golf, itself, is physical and mental therapy.

They said that I was, am handicapped. And that's a matter of interpretation and definition. Maybe that's why I chose golf. Golf has handicaps and indexes, based on ability. So if I had to play the game on crutches, I could still make it work. If I couldn't see, others could watch for me and if I couldn't walk to the ball, there are teammates to do the walking.

In other games of sport, handicaps are more personal, like playing in a wheelchair or even with artificial limbs. But, to a true sportsman, adversity is only a challenge to do something better, and sports teach values and good character and selflessness and the necessity of working together as a team. Even playing alone, you're still part of a team — the team of human beings. Sports teach decision-making and self-reliance. A handicap only makes the results more rewarding.

However, it wouldn't have hurt any to have learned to play golf before all of this happened.

CHAPTER THIRTY
"The Happiest Place On Earth"
(Disneyland, 1973)

Throughout this book, I've written about the many problems that come with this new territory and how I managed to resolve them. It took a good while. This whole process also corrected me and evolved a new person.

And, there was a method. A method is needed for organization and results — remember Chapter 10? That method was to examine my life to whatever point, concentrate on what I had been, weigh beliefs, actions and decisions of whatever problem or question against the results (taking the time for trial and error) and try to analyze their merits for me and anyone else involved. Thus the problems became those opportunities and resolving them opened the door to a new and improved version of me.

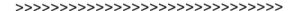

Motivation? With each situation I asked myself some hard and, importantly, honest questions and demanded of myself hard and honest answers:

✓ *Were my motives and actions selfish and juvenile or mature and adult?*

- ✓ Responsible?
- ✓ Taking or giving?
- ✓ Participating in and with life?
- ✓ Giving value for value received?
- ✓ Profitable, for me and for others?
- ✓ Was I a productive member of society?
- ✓ Can my experiences be of value to others?

Sound too goody-two-shoes? Too much like a saint? I'm not one. But I found that if I didn't try for the top, push for the best, I'd never get anywhere. I discovered that I owed life. I owed because I learned that one can't just buy life by throwing money at it. I had to work with it. Nurture it. Cultivate it. Make it grow and bear fruit. Make it mean something for those who follow and would otherwise be left to find their way alone. I had to just reach out and up, extend myself a little more. I found that feeling sorry for myself just didn't "cut it," because when my legs and feet didn't work too well, I put myself in the place of the man who had no legs, no feet. There's always someone with something more of whatever , more adversity, and if I wanted to be better, I could make it better. It's really not that hard.

As a result, a lot changed for me:
- ✓ My view of life
- ✓ My way of life
- ✓ My ability to cope with life
- ✓ My attitude toward others and myself

Now, a word or two for you, the reader (I'm not preaching, I'm just listing the facts that I learned through years of trial and error).

✓ Pessimism can destroy you. Optimism is your best friend. Don't wallow in hurt and pity, let the circumstances motivate and guide your actions. Mistakes are better than doing nothing. Besides, you learn from those mistakes.

✓ If you don't hope, believe, battle, reach out and always up — you'll never make it.

✓ Good guys finish first, not last. It just takes longer.

✓ There are going to be long and boring, frustrating days of recuperation, times of ups and downs. During that time you'll often think: why, why live and for what?

✓ Because there are lots of reasons, for you and the others around and close to you. Think of them, they've been involved, too. They've had to sacrifice, their lives in turmoil, often turned upside down. Their efforts warrant recognition and grateful thanks.

✓ You've been willing to work hard, think hard, fight hard. You've been tried by despair and disaster and disappointment — and, you've won.

✓ You feel pretty good about yourself because what you've done is quite an achievement. Don't overdo it. Maybe some others won't understand, but that's their problem. Don't hide what you are, what you think, just do it quietly in an adult and responsible way, at the proper time. You'll know.

✓ Think — I did. I am. So I can do and I

will do!

This is a story with no end. It's the saga of one life, yet of all life. Is "recovery" ever complete? I've returned to a normal life. What's normal? I'm just thankful for what is, and I know it can only get better.

And it does.

CHAPTER THIRTY-ONE
"Good To The Last Drop"
(Maxwell House Coffee, 1926, and originally coined by Theodore Roosevelt in 1907)

Time has been an ally. I adjusted, I bent, I didn't break. I took care of each difficulty as it consciously presented itself. I began to ignore what I had been but used the past as a reference, lived with it, profited and grew. As my mind, my actions adjusted to life, the energy and competitiveness necessary for the thoughtful and practical process of living and being, returned. There was always time to do it right and I let the situation be the guide.

In the very beginnings of this story we noted that it was common belief that brain cells do not, cannot regenerate themselves and other parts of the brain take over the functions.

And I began to think:

It's probably impossible for remaining portions of a totally devastated brain to assume all the complications, the functions of human existence. Just as time and proper treatment can repair other parts of the body — veins, arteries, nerves, organs, why not the brain? Scientists have discovered that heart cells regenerate. They're similar. There are many, many cells in the brain. How many were destroyed? They said the whole brain. Were some merely damaged?

Repairable, to return to function?   Do others learn new functions? A combination?

The answers to these questions are this story.

I am functioning now, much as before. Pressure and fatigue wear more easily. I'm older. The mind has been tempered with the experiences of hurt, disaster and adversity and shaped by the realities of this world. But it was molded and bent by the needs for a better existence, for myself and those loved ones who sacrificed and suffered so much. Small wonder I view this whole process as "a stroke of good luck."

And I came to the conclusion earlier than most scientific and medical professionals: brain cells must and do regenerate. It just takes time, patience and guts. How else to explain the slow, steady progress of re-growing abilities, re-growing functions, re-growing the mental to match the physical? That I'm alive. That I'm here. That I can write these words, maybe even philosophize a bit here and there, brings only one conclusion: brain cells can and do regenerate.

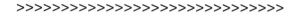

To give medical substance, let's turn back the clock.

For decades, medical science believed that the brain was a fixed object, and you were born with so many brain cells and that was that – once they died, they were gone forever and no change was possible. Fortunately, that's not true. That's not the end. Not any more.

In the early 1900s, the same Nobel Prize winner who pronounced this cruel standard in the first part of his research diagnosis also provided hope in the second part of this declaration when he stated that it was up to scientists of the future to change this harsh prognosis.

And they have.

In 1998, a scientific team in Sweden identified the creation of new cells in the adult human brain and these new cells (neural stem cells) proceeded through the Rostral Migratory Stream (RMS) to those parts of the brain that needed repair. On a separate issue, in 2002, biologists in California found this same passageway full of proliferating cells (not just a few but some 10,000 at different stages of development) and that Stream seemed to be full of growth liquids to aid in the process. And, just recently, in December of 2010, after eight years of collaborative research, scientists from New Zealand and those same pioneers from Sweden, officially confirmed this passageway and published the finding that they had found adult neural stem cells in the process of differentiating into neurons and that these neurons then traveled this RMS to repair and replace injured and dead cells in the brain.

Medicine calls it Neurogenesis.

I call it nature's damage control.

I'm no medical authority but I could see where all this was going – and, it's exciting. Just think of the potential, new ways to see and treat, not just stroke, but Alzheimers, cerebral palsy, dementia, Parkinsons, autism, more.

And, it confirms — why me, why this story,

this book, this handbook of hope. Yes, my brain repaired, re-grew and relearned to react and function to life and it's situations. I had to learn through trail and error how to rewire, retrain and re-grow my brain and my body. To control my actions and reactions and to make it all work. They call the brain plastic and the study and method is called Neuroplasticity. It's physical therapy combined with mental therapy. Yes, the brain's plastic.

I call it all just using common sense and learning how to live.

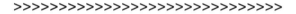

I've used up some 45,000 words sharing my experiences and thoughts, and hopefully, wisdom, with you. Perhaps it's appropriate to share what someone else had to say about these events.

My son, Richard, although very young when I had the stroke, has seen, shared in it all. Here's what he wrote about the matter for a school assignment many years ago:

"My father is a hard-working, young-looking man who has been working ever since I can remember. He is about 5'll" tall, weighs about 165, has dark brown hair and is very well dressed and clean. He had a stroke at the age of 38, but you couldn't tell it by the looks of him. The only way you can tell is by the way he acts when he is tired. He also can't control the left side of his body too well. Or, when his emotions show. When he is tired or not feeling well, little things will bother him which wouldn't bother anyone else, but what I notice most is how he has put it in his past and how he doesn't mind to talk about it. I was about six years old when he had the stroke. He was in all kinds of hospitals for three months. I could never see him or talk to him. When he got back home he didn't know who I was or even my sisters. He could barely talk, write or walk. His left side was almost paralyzed. My mom had to help him do everything. She said it was like teaching a little kid. But he remembers quickly. After a couple of months he was doing some things himself. After one and a half years he went to get his job back. They wouldn't give it to him. They said he couldn't handle it. So he got a new job and we moved nearby. He looks good. He leads a normal life like everyone else. He still has a bad temper but he has learned to control it. He still acts much the same now as he did before the stroke. He likes cars, football and all of us."

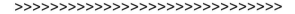

There's an old Japanese saying: Fall down seven times, get up eight. I got up. I'm still here to do things and do them better and make living mean something. To fulfill the opportunity I have been granted.

You can do as well, and probably better.

Just remember, it's not just how you handle something, it's what you do with how you handle it that counts.

Life is a gift — savor it, nourish it, help it grow.

THE BEGINNING